PRACTISING WELFARE RIGHTS

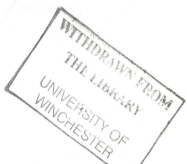

Practising Welfare Rights aims to improve awareness among people working in social work and advice agencies about the skills required for effective welfare rights work, and offers guidance for managers and other professionals about how to develop a welfare rights service.

Written by a well-known author, trainer and adviser on welfare rights issues, this book includes:

- learning objectives
- activities to test understanding
- illustrative case studies

It also covers core welfare rights skills, such as interviewing, legal research, negotiation and advocacy, and discusses the historical, social and economic forces which have shaped welfare rights practice as well as the politics of welfare.

An accessible book which highlights the place of welfare rights practice in modern society, *Practising Welfare Rights* is essential reading for welfare rights and other advice workers, social workers and social care practitioners, professionals and managers in social work and welfare rights settings and anyone studying social work.

Neil Bateman is an internationally renowned author, trainer and consultant specialising in welfare rights and social policy issues. His articles have been frequently published in the social care and public services press. Previous books include *Advocacy Skills for Health and Social Care Professionals* (2000), and contributions to a number of welfare rights and social work reference books. More information can be found at **www.neilbateman.co.uk**

the social work skills series

published in association with *Community Care*

series editor: Terry Philpot, Editor-in-Chief

the social work skills series

- builds practice skills step by step
- places practice in its policy context
- relates practice to relevant research
- provides a secure base for professional development

This new, skills-based series has been developed by Routledge and *Community Care* working together in partnership to meet the changing needs of today's students and practitioners in the broad field of social care. Written by experienced practitioners and teachers with a commitment to passing on their knowledge to the next generation, each text in the series features: *learning objectives; case examples; activities to test knowledge and understanding; summaries of key learning points; key references; suggestions for further reading.*

Also available in the series:

Commissioning and Purchasing
Terry Bamford
Former Chair of the British Association of Social Workers and Executive Director of Housing and Social Services, Royal Borough of Kensington and Chelsea.

Managing Aggression
Ray Braithwaite
Consultant and trainer in managing aggression at work. Lead trainer and speaker in the 'No Fear' campaign.

Tackling Social Exclusion
John Pierson
Senior Lecturer at the Institute of Social Work and Applied Social Studies at the University of Staffordshire.

Safeguarding Children and Young People
Corinne May-Chahal and Stella Coleman
Professor of Applied Social Science at Lancaster University.
Senior Lecturer in Social Work at the University of Central Lancashire.

The Task-Centred Book
Mark Doel and Peter Marsh
Research Professor of Social Work at Sheffield Hallam University.
Professor of Child and Family Welfare, University of **Sheffield**.

Practising Welfare Rights
Neil Bateman
Author, trainer and consultant specialising in welfare rights and social policy issues.

Using Groupwork
Mark Doel
Research Professor of Social Work at Sheffield Hallam University

PRACTISING WELFARE RIGHTS

Neil Bateman

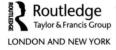
Routledge
Taylor & Francis Group

LONDON AND NEW YORK

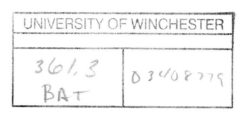

First published 2006 by Routledge
2 Park Square, Milton Park, Abingdon, Oxon OX14 4RN

Simultaneously published in the USA and Canada
by Routledge
270 Madison Ave, New York, NY 10016

Routledge is an imprint of the Taylor and Francis Group

© 2006 Neil Bateman
The right of Neil Bateman to be identified as author of this work has been
asserted by him in accordance with the Copyright Design and Patents Act 1988

Designed and typeset in Sabon and Futura by
Keystroke, Jacaranda Lodge, Wolverhampton
Printed and bound in Great Britain by
TJ International Ltd, Padstow, Cornwall

British Library Cataloguing in Publication Data
A catalogue record for this book is available from the British Library

Library of Congress Cataloging in Publication Data
A catalog record for this book has been requested

ISBN10: 0–415–35889–2 (hbk)
ISBN10: 0–415–35890–6 (pbk)

ISBN13: 9–78–0–415–35889–7 (hbk)
ISBN13: 9–78–0–415–35890–3 (pbk)

CONTENTS

PREFACE

Welfare rights practice is a hugely empowering and exciting way of helping people. It has been part of my life since the early 1970s, when I started as a young activist in a claimants union while a law student. Since then, the impact of a successful welfare rights case on the quality of life of the individual still amazes me and constantly reaffirms that it is a legitimate and essential tool in today's world.

Since my student days, welfare rights practice has become mainstreamed in many ways but retains the status of an outsider activity. This is both a strength and a weakness.

This book partly came about as a result of my own faith in welfare rights practice as something unique and valuable and which has a role both in challenging abuses of power by officialdom and as a small step in redressing the huge inequalities in the UK today.

I have tried to write this book in a way which makes it relevant to both welfare rights specialists and those with an interest in welfare rights work, but who are non-specialists. I also look at some of the strategic issues facing welfare rights practitioners and offer some advice about how to develop a welfare rights service. It is not a technical handbook (there are already many good ones available), but is a book about nothing more and nothing less than the practice of welfare rights advice and advocacy.

ACKNOWLEDGEMENTS

I hesitate to start a book which aims to be accessible by referring to a political philosopher, but it is relevant. John Rawls argued that individual achievement is a myth and that any individual success was due to the efforts of many others and of society as a whole by supporting, helping and providing resources to an individual.

I may be the person who types it all out on a keyboard, but my work on this book is not mine alone and it would not have been possible without the help, advice and support of many people, including people in several countries. Their generosity with their time and their expertise has turned what would otherwise have been a dry and narrow book into one which takes in history, geography, socio-legal policy and global politics.

I would therefore like to place on record my sincere thanks to all the following who have helped and who are listed in no particular order.

Terry Philpot, my commissioning editor, Gary Vaux of Hertfordshire County Council Money Advice Unit and Geoff Fimister, anti-poverty consultant in Newcastle, for reading and commenting on drafts and other help, Peter Young, Social Security Attorney of Mill Valley in California, for also commenting on drafts, John Bouman at the Sargent Shriver Poverty Law Center in Chicago, John Freedman from New York's Welfare Law Center, Colin Daly of Northside (Coolock) Community Law Centre in Dublin and Robert Lynch of the Irish National Organisation for the Unemployed, Daniel Spagni from the Advanced Research Partnership at Manchester University, Gill Terry, Claire Tolliday and Jo Cowley from Suffolk County Council's Financial Inclusion and Advice Service, Michael Raper of the Welfare Rights Centre in Sydney, Australia, Will Somerville latterly of Inclusion and now at the Commission for Racial Equality, Paul Bivand and Liz Britton from Inclusion, Bonnie Thompson in British Columbia, Canada, David Mossop QC of the Community Legal Assistance Society in Vancouver, Canada, Marge Reitsma-Street at Victoria University in Canada, Jon Pierson, Duncan Tree of Community Service Volunteers, Rita Davies of London Borough of Newham Social Regeneration Unit, Aaron Barbour from Community Links Trust in east London, Katherine Hickey of Free Legal Advice Centres Ireland, my father-in-law Clunie Dale, former Trades Union Congress Social Insurance Secretary, staff at the German Advice Centre in London, Carol O'Byrne of Cardiff City Council Welfare Rights Service, Calum MacKinnon of North Lanarkshire Council Welfare Rights Service, Alban Hawksworth of Age Concern England, Andy Pennington of South London and Maudsley NHS Trust,

Dr Jean Adams of the School of Population and Health Sciences University of Newcastle upon Tyne Medical School, Delyth Owens of Citizens Advice Cymru, Novello Maynard-Thompson of Ipswich for his poetry, Sarah Sanford and Mary Hughes from Ipswich Community Resource Centre, Jacqueline Davidson from the University of Stirling and Sarah Collins from Middlesbrough Council's Welfare Rights Service.

And finally, of course, Julie, Jessica, Caitlin and Calum.

My genuine apologies if I have missed out anyone.

Neil Bateman, Ipswich, Suffolk, United Kingdom, May 2005
www.neilbateman.co.uk

CLAIMING INCOME SUPPORT

Novello Maynard-Thompson

Anyone claiming Income Support will be debased by the rules,
It does not mean the people claiming it are classified as fools,
The amount of money saved you can have is too petty a sum
The most brilliant of claimant can see that even classed as rum.

It will not buy new your household comforts only second hand stuff,
If on it long term you become like the cheap goods – a bit of fluff,
What you have saved affects your housing benefit allowed for rent,
Either agree to the rules or buy yourself a second hand tent.

The way forwards for all us claimants could be identity card,
As long as no-one remains homeless and have to sleep in the yard.

© 2005 Novello Maynard-Thompson

Novello Maynard-Thompson lives in Ipswich and is a poet, musician and artist who has experienced the social security system and mental health services.

CHAPTER 1

WHAT IS WELFARE RIGHTS PRACTICE?

OBJECTIVES

By the end of this chapter you should:

▪ Understand the essential nature of welfare rights practice

▪ Know about the history of welfare rights activity

▪ Have some knowledge about welfare rights provision in some countries outside the UK

▪ Understand the role and development of welfare rights practice in relation to government economic and social policy.

A ROUGH DEFINITION

> Welfare rights work aims to maximise service users' social security income by giving them information and advice and advocating on their behalf; advocacy is particularly employed when a benefit has been denied.
>
> (Bateman in Davies 2000: 370)

Welfare rights practice features to a greater or lesser extent in the daily work of many public sector and voluntary agency workers (the helping services) who have contact with people living on a low income. There are also advice workers and some lawyers who specialise in welfare rights work, often taking referrals from people working in the helping services. These advisers are usually based in local government or the voluntary sector but occasionally can be found in the private sector.

EXAMPLES OF WELFARE RIGHTS PRACTICE

Welfare rights practice covers a diverse range of activity around the benefits system. Some welfare rights activities require tremendous technical skills and knowledge, others can be carried out by people whose main work does not include welfare rights practice. The key is to distinguish which type of work falls into different skill levels.

The following are examples of welfare rights practice:

- checking whether someone is receiving all the benefits they are entitled to
- helping to complete a claim form for disability living allowance
- making a supersession request for someone on attendance allowance whose health has deteriorated in order to increase the amount of benefit they receive
- helping someone to appeal against a refusal of benefit
- advising someone about how to deal with a medical examination in connection with a benefit claim
- obtaining evidence to help support a claim
- advising about conditions of entitlement for someone who is subject to immigration control
- obtaining an interim payment of benefit where there is a delay in processing a benefit claim
- advising about the implications of doing voluntary work or studying while receiving Jobseeker's Allowance
- calculating whether or not someone will be better off if they take a low paid job after receiving means-tested benefits
- challenging a benefit or tax credit overpayment
- monitoring poor customer service by a benefits provider, assembling the evidence and lobbying for improvements
- writing a letter setting out why someone qualifies for backdated benefit.

While welfare rights specialists may also have skills and knowledge in a number of related areas such as housing rights, debt, immigration law and community care rights, welfare rights is primarily concerned with rights to income from the state. The name has its origins in the USA, where the word 'welfare' is used colloquially to refer to the US means-tested benefits system (as opposed to 'social security' in the USA, which refers to the well-established and parallel system of income maintenance based on compulsory insurance contributions). In the UK, 'welfare rights' covers both means-tested and non-means-tested benefits.

The growth of debt among those on low incomes in recent years and the worsening of debt by benefit problems, by state administered usury in the shape of Social Fund loans, administrative failure and general benefit underclaiming means that there are often common skills and knowledge among both debt and welfare rights advisers. However, the issue is clouded by the preponderance of poorly regulated private companies offering debt advice, usually earning money from lending or debt settlement. A large number of non-specialists working within the welfare state will also undertake debt advice and advocacy to some extent. With nearly half of all lone parents and a quarter of couple families in arrears with regular commitments, debt advice and advocacy are frequent companions to welfare rights advice. And welfare rights advice and advocacy are often key components in addressing an individual's debts. However, the skills and knowledge involved in debt advice are a specialism in their own right and this area of work has its own history, so I do not discuss them in this book.

Compared to many other types of activity undertaken by people in the helping services, welfare rights practice is unique because its main focus is on the worker acting as an advocate for the service user (also known as 'client', 'claimant' or 'customer') and with challenging negative decisions on benefit entitlement. As a result, welfare rights practice has a strong, if unwritten, ethical basis concerned with pursuing the client's rights. Welfare rights practice without such an ethical basis is an activity which is more characteristic of benefits administration or simple information giving and should not be described as welfare rights activity.

What marks out welfare rights practice from other work involving advice on benefits is its rights perspective. The way we give advice, how we interpret rights and what we do to help people achieve them will be closely linked to the values of the organisation we work for or our own personal values – advice giving is not a value-free or neutral activity. This means that one of the hallmarks of welfare rights practice is that it is independent of the agency being advocated against, otherwise there is always going to be a conflict of interest. Local authorities which also administer housing benefit and council tax benefit have usually agreed protocols to safeguard the ability of their own in-house welfare rights service and staff working in other services to advise and advocate on housing and council tax benefit issues. There is also legal authority for the acceptability of staff in one part of a local authority to act as advocates against the local authority's own benefits service: in Social Security and Child Support Commissioner's decision CH 729/03 it was held that there was no fatal conflict of interest in a local authority welfare rights officer's representation of a housing benefit claimant in dispute with that officer's employing authority, but that good practice was to make the relationship clear to the appellant, ideally with provision for the latter to confirm in writing that this had been explained.

The issue of independence is discussed further in Chapter 2 – particularly in the light of recent moves to reduce organisational barriers between the Department for Work and Pensions (DWP) and other bodies.

BOX 1.1:   SKILLS USED IN WELFARE RIGHTS PRACTICE

The skills used in welfare rights practice include:

- interviewing and listening
- record keeping
- managing time and self
- researching the law and sometimes a service user's social, family and medical circumstances
- clarifying key, relevant facts in real life situations
- interpreting legislation and guidance and applying them to those facts
- improving skills associated with self-development
- keeping up-to-date with changes and developments in social security and related areas
- presenting the best case – orally and/or in writing
- utilising persuasion skills combined with a rights-based and legal approach (for more skilled welfare rights practitioners, this includes being able to do so at tribunals and other appellate bodies)
- developing assertiveness and tenacity (not being fearful of authority and being able to pursue a case to achieve a satisfactory result for the service user)
- being able to know when one has reached one's limits, seeking help and asking for a second opinion and if need be, knowing when to let go
- having transparent, efficient and mutually agreed referral arrangements to more skilled advisers
- developing skills in campaigning and lobbying to secure improvements to the benefits system
- having skills in publicity and promotion to encourage and help people who are on a low income but who are underclaiming to make successful benefit claims.

ACTIVITY 1.1

Consider how the skills listed above are also relevant to other areas of your daily life and/or work.

SOME PHILOSOPHICAL ASPECTS

A welfare rights approach reflects broader socio-economic changes and the development of formal welfare and income maintenance systems since the Second World War. Welfare rights are also a sign of wider social rights and the campaigns to achieve these which in western countries have their origins in the pre-war years and the realisation during the Second World War that while democratic and other civil rights had largely been achieved, rights to health, housing, education and freedom from poverty were yet to be realised.

As well as putting the relationship between the individual and the state on a more equal footing and ensuring proper accountability of state activity, rights to welfare reflect the move away from income maintenance systems based on paternalism or complete discretion rooted in subjective notions of deservedness. They reflect the development of more mature social security systems founded upon the rule of law rather than charitable values. This means that detailed rules about who does or does not qualify have had to be developed and in turn these increase the scope for debates about entitlement and the need for impartial adjudication of disputes. In the UK, the growth of means-testing in the social security system, especially since the 1980s (a process accelerated by Tony Blair's governments, particularly with the introduction of pension credit and tax credits), has inevitably meant that it has been necessary to have a parallel growth in the particularly complex types of rules which determine means-tested benefit entitlement.

The period since 1988 has also seen a noticeable trend of developing state income maintenance without formal appeal rights and this has accelerated under the Blair governments – this is discussed further in Chapter 2.

Dean (2002: 7) has written extensively about the development of rights and social welfare and summarises one approach to rights by writers on legal philosophy as follows: 'Rights are created by rules that benefit the human individual by imposing obligations upon other individuals to protect or further her interests'. However, Dean suggests that this definition fails to adequately reflect the historical origins of welfare rights (being founded on collective pressure and campaigning by people living in poverty and their advocates). Dean (2002) also examines how the nature of welfare rights will vary according to the type of welfare system that exists in a country. So, for example, countries with income maintenance systems which are more minimalist (such as the USA) will have a different view of welfare rights than those with a more universal system (such as Denmark).

HISTORY OF WELFARE RIGHTS MOVEMENTS AND SOME INTERNATIONAL PERSPECTIVES

Welfare rights work is not new and has been around for a long time. There is clear evidence of an advocacy role being adopted by, for example, workers employed by the British nineteenth-century Charity Organisation Society (the first documented social workers) to press for charitable grants and Poor Law relief for individuals and families. Sidney and Beatrice Webb, who broke away from the society in search of a more radical approach, clearly saw themselves as advocates. Thus the social work profession's earliest days embedded the concept of social workers as advocates on welfare rights and income maintenance issues. This was reflected in the writings of early pioneers such as Mary Richmond (1917) and Charlotte Towle (1945), who emphasised the need for income maximisation as part of the social work task; the advocacy involved in 'obtaining relief' was a legitimate part of their role.

Similarly, in Canada, before the implementation of formal social security systems in the 1940s, the work of members of each province's legislative assembly included pressing for financial help for individuals from each province's indigent funds. As the funds being applied for in both the UK and Canada were charitable and/or discretionary, the advocate would rely on making a 'worthy' case, rather than persuasion based on interpretation of rules, as would occur with advocacy involving a benefits system based on legal rules.

The foundations of the modern UK income maintenance system were laid by the Liberal governments of Henry Campbell-Bannerman and Herbert Asquith, particularly under the influence of David Lloyd George, when he was Chancellor of the Exchequer in the period after 1908, culminating in the National Insurance Act 1911. The reforms of that era provided at least basic income maintenance for pensioners aged 70 or older (not such a large group at that time, given early death rates) and some unemployed people. These reforms were part of a larger collection of social reforms which the then Liberal government adopted, though compulsory insurance for workers disabled through work-related accidents dates back to the 1890s and the first health and safety legislation was in 1871.

The UK's social security reforms were actually comparatively late, with the first developments of a more universal social security system being found in Otto von Bismarck's reforms of 1883–1889, followed by Austria in 1888, and Italy and Switzerland in the 1890s. Bismarck's reforms may well have been motivated by a desire to outmanoeuvre his leftist opponents and reinforce the unification of Germany but they displayed some surprisingly modern and universalist features, with worker representation on schemes administering benefits, the sweeping away of charitable and parish-based approaches (which the UK did not complete until 1948) and providing coverage for a large percentage of the population (Thomson 1966: 358).

The codification of rights required the development of a system to adjudicate claims which had been turned down and an appeals system was developed which opened the way for people to act as advocates using an approach based on interpretation of rules.

However, even before this, the history books show that the UK's old Poor Law system, with its emphasis on locally determined and provided relief, discretion and usually harshness, could be challenged by collective and/or legal action. For example, the case of *West Ham v Owens (1872) (36 J.P. 776)* (Moss 1938: 64) involved a legal challenge to the powers of the local parish to recover the cost of Poor Law relief from someone who had been a beneficiary. There was also social reformer Louisa Twining, who went on to form the Workhouse Visiting Society. It is thought that she was involved in petitioning on behalf of individuals in the Strand and other workhouses (Higginbotham 2005).

However, instances of formal advocacy appear to be unusual and help explain the injustices brought about by the use of unbridled prejudice and power by the Boards of Guardians and Relieving Officers who administered Poor Law relief and the workhouses. Consequently, even today, some older people still have a sense of humiliation when claiming means-tested benefits; 'you work all your life and then you end up facing a means test' is a common refrain.

During the 1930s there were documented examples of welfare rights advocacy in the UK by groups such as the National Unemployed Workers Movement. Not only did they represent individual claimants who had been refused unemployment benefits (usually because of the application of the very harsh means test between 1931 and 1935), but also they undertook benefit take-up campaigns, helping people to claim benefits which they were entitled to, frequently to the annoyance of the officials administering these benefits by presenting themselves with groups of destitute unemployed people at Labour Exchanges. Apparently in Chesterfield in 1929, angered by the cutting-off of benefits to unemployed people who could not prove they were 'genuinely seeking employment' by not having their 'green cards' signed by employers, 3,000 jobless people presented themselves en masse at a local factory asking for individual written confirmation of jobseeking by having their green cards signed. This type of action was not uncommon and was deliberately aimed at not only ridiculing but also making it impossible to operate such punitive systems (Merton Claimants Action Group 2004).

During the 1940s the first Citizens Advice Bureaux were established in order to provide information and advice to people affected by events in the Second World War. They soon began to establish themselves as a national network of advice agencies and independent advice and advocacy on benefits was part of their advice services during this period. In 1948, legislation was passed which brought about the legal aid scheme to provide free or low cost legal advice to people on low incomes and of course also at this time, the more familiar shape of the UK's income maintenance system was established (though the Poor Law system had been in decline since the Unemployment Assistance Board was established in 1937 and evolved into the Assistance Board in 1940).

The 1950s and 1960s were characterised by persistent low unemployment with high demand for low skill labour, low inflation for most of this era and lower levels of wealth inequality than have been the case since the 1980s. Poverty as a political issue became very marginal compared to the 1930s and 1940s (for example, when the Beveridge Report proposing the establishment of a comprehensive welfare state was published in 1942, long queues formed outside the publishers and people in the armed forces had briefings and debates about it). The then Prime Minister Harold Macmillan's line in a 1957 speech that 'most of our people have never had it so good' is frequently seen as a fair reflection of the collective political view of poverty in this era.

As well as improved economic conditions, the benefits system in this period was characterised by historically low numbers claiming means-tested benefits (principally national assistance) and non-means-tested, national insurance social security benefits which were often higher in real terms than they are today. From the perspective of benefit statistics, life in the 1950s certainly looked rosy. In 1950 just 77,000 people received national assistance (the forerunner of supplementary benefit introduced in 1966, thence replaced by income support in 1988), remaining below 100,000 until 1958. The numbers then increased slowly but even by the start of 1965, just 112,000 people depended on national assistance. By comparison, in 2003, the numbers on income support had reached 3.96 million (source: Policy Studies Institute/Department for Work and Pensions), a figure set to grow with the increase of pension credit in October 2003 and tax credits which all have means-tested eligibility criteria that broaden entitlement to ever greater proportions of the population.

The period from 1962 to 1965 was characterised by the phenomenon dubbed the 'rediscovery of poverty', which was prompted by the writing and research of social scientists such as Peter Townsend, Brian Abel-Smith and later Tony Lynes as well as numerous non-academic writers who cast doubt on the alleged success of the post-war welfare state's success in eliminating poverty and who highlighted the inadequate scope and level of benefits.

The rediscovery of poverty not only had an influence on government policy but also strongly helped the founding of new campaigning organisations such as Shelter, the Child Poverty Action Group and the Disability Alliance. There was also frustration among activists in the 1960s about Harold Wilson's Labour government's social policies:

> Labour went to the hustings in 1964 behind a rhetoric of science and modernisation that served to both unite the party in the wake of Gaitskell's death, and to express in a highly ambiguous fashion the Wilson leadership's overriding priorities of economic growth, a strong currency and an inter-ventionist state. Increasingly, Harold Wilson's emphasis on the 'white heat of the technological revolution' came to displace the 1959 theme of closing the gap between rich and poor. Wilson's highly administrative style of politics, and his preoccupation with the theme of economic growth as the prerequisite for social action had convinced many Labour activists that an initiative in the welfare field must perforce come from outside the party leadership.
>
> (McCarthy 1986: 39)

One can of course also see parallels with frustration with New Labour in the 2000s.

Child Poverty Action Group (CPAG), founded in 1965, has become perhaps foremost among organisations in the UK welfare rights field, providing technical and policy support to people engaged in welfare rights work, pursuing test cases and lobbying government. However, it was not founded as a welfare rights organisation per se and developed welfare rights advocacy as a result of publicising the problem of poor take-up of benefit entitlement and being asked by individual claimants for help with benefit problems from about 1967 onwards (see D. Bull in Curtis and Sanderson 2004: 116). The US Civil Rights and Welfare Rights movements also strongly influenced CPAG's approach.

BORN IN THE USA?

In the USA, the early to late 1960s saw a change in political campaigning because of the impact of the Civil Rights Movement. The scale and depth of poverty among African Americans, particularly in the southern states, exacerbated by discriminatory and arbitrary application of welfare rules by white officials and judgemental use of discretion by individual states, led to the development of what is now known as welfare rights work to help people achieve what they were entitled to, to lobby for improvement in welfare provision and to improve take-up of benefits. The scale of poverty among African Americans, and the sheer injustice of the welfare system they dealt with, meant that welfare rights activity had to be a key element of any struggle for equal treatment on racial grounds. '[welfare] rules as written were laden with cultural and class biases about what constituted proper motherhood and acceptable personal behaviour' (Nadasen 2005: 48). While it came to prominence during the 1960s and did eventually go on to receive federal funding, the US welfare rights movement can be traced back to the 1950s, being based around groups of welfare recipients organising collectively to challenge capricious practices, raise awareness of rights and to lobby for improvements. However, the alliance in the 1960s between these activists, the Civil Rights Movement and radical lawyers led to their era of greatest prominence. So much so that by this time over 100,000 welfare recipients were members of welfare rights organisations in the USA.

The National Coordinating Committee of Welfare Rights Groups was established in 1966 with many of the locally based groups receiving substantial public funding under the benign influence of politicians like Democrat Vice President Hubert Humphrey and as part of the then Democrat Administration's War on Poverty dating back to 1964 and influenced by the USA's own rediscovery of poverty through the introduction of its Poverty Index in 1959.

A number of important test cases were successful. One example (which seems incredible by today's standards) was the victory in the US Supreme Court (equivalent in judicial terms to the House of Lords in the UK) to enable children in Alabama to receive welfare when their mother was living with a man whom she was not married to (*King v Smith 392 U.S. 309 (1968)*) by applying the supremacy of federal law over state law. Alabama had developed discriminatory regulations about Aid to Dependent Families with Children (ADFC). These were struck down as inconsistent with the federal legislation which provided the funding for Alabama's ADFC programme. Another was the Supreme Court's decision to give welfare recipients the right to a fair hearing before cutting off their income (*Goldberg v Kelly 397 U.S. 254 (1970)*) because of safeguards in the US constitution (Bailey and Brake 1975: 118; Nadasen 2005: 60). The Goldberg case was a particular landmark and was progressed in conjunction with a mass public campaign. Hence the influence of the USA on the UK's welfare rights movement.

Nowadays welfare rights activity in the USA appears to fall into several categories which reflects the fragmented nature of the US social security and welfare systems and of course there is no equivalent of the UK's free National Health Service, with help towards medical costs coming from the Medicare and means-tested Medicaid schemes.

The US benefits system includes comparatively generous social insurance benefits for old age, disability and survivors (the Old-Age Survivors and Disability Insurance Program or 'Title II benefits') which date back to Roosevelt's New Deal and the Social Security Act 1935, means-tested supplemental security income ('Title XVI benefits') paid at lower rates for elders, and people with a disability who have incomplete social insurance records, Temporary Aid to Needy Families (TANF) introduced as part of the 1996 welfare reforms which President Bill Clinton acceded to under Republican pressure. These generally provide up to five years' means-tested help to people with children as well as the Food Stamp Program. TANF replaced Aid to Dependent Families with Children, which was also part of the Roosevelt reforms. The Clinton reforms mark a watershed in welfare policy which has reached across the Atlantic and which have huge implications for anyone working in the welfare state nowadays. A pre-occupation among rightwing commentators (such as found in Charles Murray's 1984 book *Losing Ground: American Social Policy 1950–1980*), that welfare allegedly undermined society gained credibility in the Ronald Reagan years and despite the lack of objective evidence to support the views, statements such as welfare 'erodes work and family and thus keeps poor people poor' (George Gilder cited in Tree 1999) have become widely acceptable and accepted.

The new right's influence in the USA (deepened by George W. Bush's favouring of fundamentalist Christian welfare institutions and his administration's refusal to engage with welfare lobbyists who do not share this perspective) has a pervasive influence on UK politicians across the parties. The dismantling and undermining of welfare provision in the USA has also been made easier by the split responsibilities between states and the federal government and the historically general reluctance of federal government to be seen as championing welfare (Tree 1999: 13). Would this arise in the UK if aspects of social security were devolved to Northern Ireland, Wales and Scotland?

Many groups experience difficulty accessing benefits in the USA – for example, advocacy has been undertaken by the New York Welfare Law Center to challenge apparently deliberate delays and unlawful overscrutiny of applications for TANF and Food Stamps. Another recent example is the class action by the Chicago-based Sargent Shriver National Center on Poverty Law about the underprovision of Medicaid to low income children by the state of Illinois (*Memisovski et al. v Meram* F.Supp.2d *(N.D.Ill., 2004)*). A similar principle was successfully applied to challenge Pennsylvania's lack of Medicaid funding of dental care in *Clark v Richman (No 4:00-CV-1306 (2003))*, a case supported by the National Senior Citizens Law Center.

Social security advocates have also broadened the scope of Title II benefits through their input to many of the 996,000 appeals against negative decisions (a very high appeal to claim ratio of 40 per cent: US Social Security Administration 2005).

Current welfare rights services in the USA include the following:

- About 4,000 attorneys and non-attorney advocates in private practice are members of the National Organisation of Social Security Claimants Representatives, who provide help and advocacy mostly in obtaining Title II benefits, funded by contingency fees ('No win. No pay') taking a proportion of backdated benefit and with very occasional funding from the US Legal Services Corporation. The nature of Title XVI benefits means that it is not possible to fund private attorneys, and limited federal funding for legal services leaves a huge gap, filled to an extent by local welfare agencies and support groups.

- A network of poverty and welfare law centres, funded mostly by charitable donations, provides advocacy and help primarily around access and sufficiency of TANF and Food Stamps and also access to Medicare and Medicaid. These centres will also provide advocacy on discrimination and employment issues as well as run practical programmes of training and education for people living in poverty and lobby for improvement in welfare law. Public funding from the Legal Services Corporation has been very difficult since restrictions in 1996 on public law litigation.
- Social workers in hospitals advocate and help people access Medicaid to meet their medical bills.
- Grass roots welfare rights groups organise and campaign against deficiencies in welfare provision as well as providing access to help with social welfare law problems.

IRELAND COMBATS POVERTY

The Irish social security system has traditionally been regarded as inferior to the British. While this may be true historically, it is a Brit-supremacist view that fails to recognise the changes in Ireland in recent years. In many respects the Irish benefits system provides far greater and better coverage and does not have the distinct antipathy to claimants which characterises much of the UK's system. Irish people returning to live in Ireland after working in the UK remark that they find the Irish system noticeably more user friendly and flexible than the UK's.

The implementation of the National Anti-Poverty Strategy in 1986 has brought about major changes in public welfare provision and the economic growth experienced by Ireland has funded many of the consequent changes. However, several of the positive changes in benefits have been funded by cuts elsewhere in the benefits system.

Irish social work professionals have a more ambivalent relationship to welfare rights advocacy because of their involvement with supplementary social welfare payments administered by their employing organisations, the health boards.

A significant amount of welfare rights work takes place through the network of advice and advocacy bodies – the Free Legal Advice Centres (FLAC) which take on more complex test cases, the national (government funded) Comhairle (pronounced 'corla') network of advice and advocacy services, the 20 Trade Union Centres affiliated to the Irish Congress of Trade Unions, 200 local centres and organisations affiliated to the Irish National Organisation of the Unemployed and the Citizens Information Centres (equivalent to Citizens Advice Bureaux in the UK). Government funding provides the bedrock for these organisations.

Publications by Comhairle suggest a more hesitant embracing of the advocacy role and the FLAC network provides a more robust approach to welfare rights work. FLAC was established in Ireland, initially using volunteer advisers in 1969

> at the end of a decade of rapid change in Irish and European society. A largely rural population was becoming industrialised. The Seventies, it was correctly assumed, would see major social changes. But in the arena of social rights the old Ireland rather than the new Ireland still predominated. Single pregnant women had little option but to have their babies adopted, usually in secret. Until 1974, women were obliged to leave banks and civil service employment when they married. Contraception was banned until then. There was no divorce or judicial separation and, at the time, no prospect of their introduction. A married woman could not qualify for unemployment assistance unless her husband had a disability.
>
> (O'Morain 2003: 7)

FLAC has been responsible for several significant test cases about Irish Social Welfare. These include *The State (Kershaw) v Eastern Health Board* (1985) to ensure the provision of fuel vouchers to those on short-term social welfare payments, *Cotter and McDermott v Minister for Social Welfare and Attorney General* (1991) which brought in more than €350 million in arrears of welfare payments to over 70,000 married women, and *Hyland v Minister for Social Welfare* (1989) which equalised treatment of married and unmarried couples by the benefits system (O'Morain 2003: 38).

As part of the National Anti-Poverty Strategy, Irish social security institutions have not only become concerned with improving standards and levels of benefit, but also actively developed customer care services and are reported as being 'officially' relaxed, to the point of welcoming advocacy against them by external bodies, though welfare rights advisers suggest that this is not always borne out in practice at lower levels and the need for welfare rights advocacy remains as strong as ever.

Interestingly, even nowadays there are almost no formal links or joint planning between activists in the USA, Ireland, the UK and elsewhere to develop welfare rights services and Australia, the Netherlands and Canada are other countries where parallel developments have occurred. But anyone reading material published by welfare rights and social security advocates in other countries will be struck by how similar the tone and approach are with that found in similar publications in the UK. This is not a coincidence, but neither is it a conspiracy.

THE UK'S HEAVY 1970s AND 1980s

The 1970s was a period of early consolidation for the welfare rights movement in the UK which saw it grow in influence and also develop as a strand in several areas of professional practice.

The National Federation of Claimants Unions, a grass roots led organisation also founded in the 1960s, campaigned at local and national level to highlight deficiencies in benefits rules, poor practices by benefit officials (such as about how they applied the 'cohabitation rule' by asking female claimants details about their sexual relationships) as well as to provide information, advice and representation to individual claimants. The widespread existence of discretionary rules in the then supplementary benefits scheme provided a fulcrum for much agitation and advocacy, both individual and collective. As the system became more complex, grass roots led organisations had difficulty securing funding for advice activity and greater levels of expertise and professionalism were demanded. The Claimants Unions also had a highly informal and libertarian approach to organisation which did not fare well if leading people changed and which was inevitably slow to respond to external changes. One distinctive feature of the National Federation of Claimants Unions was their uncompromising view of the way the benefits system treated claimants, perhaps best summed up by their written submission to the Department of Health and Social Security's Committee on Single Parents (The 'Finer Committee', formed in 1969 and reporting in 1974). It consisted of the following statement: 'Bullshit. It's all Bullshit.' The claimant led organisations are currently neither strong nor common (unlike the USA today) – perhaps a victim of the growing professionalisation of welfare rights practice?

The early development and continued existence of active, claimant led welfare rights groups in the USA is distinct from the professional led and developed welfare rights movement in the UK. There may be many reasons for this, including the greater harshness and gaps of the US system leading to historically greater numbers of people in poverty, the tradition of community organising from the Civil Rights Movement, and the greater availability of charitable funding for such groups. In the UK, the tradition of popular organising is much more workplace based, through trade unions, and the demise of Claimants Unions has left a vacuum – though undoubtedly much of the individual advocacy undertaken by Claimants Unions is now done by paid welfare rights advocates in local authorities and voluntary agencies.

The highly discretionary nature of the supplementary benefits scheme between 1966 and its reform in 1980 provided endless injustices to challenge but it was a very simple system compared to the highly regulated successor schemes (such as income support) and it had enormous flexibility enabling even very unskilled advocates to successfully challenge refusals and/or obtain extras. As one older social care professional, who had used the scheme over the years to relieve poverty among her service users, told me: 'It wasn't perfect, but it was easy to get something for people'. I've also heard similar sentiments from former DHSS (the old Department of Health and Social Security) staff. Some of the common practices in benefits offices also readily gave people a cause – I can well remember visiting the old DHSS office in Southampton in 1974 and witnessing verbal abuse being routinely and publicly meted out to claimants by DHSS staff. Indeed, it was this particular experience which created my interest in welfare rights issues.

Having had the forerunner of the UK's first law centre open in 1967 in the shape of free legal advice sessions in Notting Hill in London, law centres continued to spread throughout the 1970s, injecting legal expertise into welfare rights advocacy and helping the development of a small cadre of solicitors and barristers with expertise in this field. In turn, an increasing number of law schools started teaching options on social welfare law as part of a conscious effort to help lawyers provide services which were more relevant to those living in poverty. Increasing numbers of social work courses began to include some teaching about welfare rights and offering practice placements which focused on welfare rights work and in some cases helping establish welfare rights advice services – such as the Oxford Community Work Organisation's Barton Advice Centre which still operates now and receives local authority funding.

Welfare rights practice has long been part of the work of social workers in the UK, even though its profile has waxed and waned over the years. The long-standing separation of cash and care in the British welfare state has been a key driver behind the acceptance of the right and ability of social workers to act as advocates on social security matters. So it is not surprising that the social work profession has contributed much to this area of practice as well as being a route into full time welfare rights work for some practitioners. However, by contrast in the USA, the involvement of many state employed social workers in income maintenance functions and the parallel provision by their employing bodies of means-tested welfare, has severely curtailed their involvement in welfare rights practice. The links between social work and welfare rights practice are discussed in more depth in Chapter 2.

With its emphasis on challenging injustices and poor benefits administration, welfare rights work inevitably became associated with the radical and socialist traditions within public services which have long promoted approaches which move welfare provision away from a charitable or paternalistic onto a more egalitarian basis. However, there were some on the left who viewed welfare rights practice critically:

> Welfare rights is a strategy that has been enthusiastically accepted across the liberal-left spectrum, and it is a seductive one for radicals for it can embody a refusal to interpret the client's view of the problem in an 'expert' way, and it gives short-term rewards of material benefit to those in poverty. It is assumed to be a good strategy, but we find in it very little discussion of the nature of poverty, how it can be changed, or the role of the state.
>
> (Bailey and Brake 1975: 113)

Three decades later it is interesting to reflect that as welfare rights practice has become a more mainstream activity in many public sector organisations, it has built on and developed the work of welfare rights bodies in the 1960s when welfare rights practice went hand-in-hand with a structural critique in key contexts and using such evidence as a methodology for criticising the state's behaviour and government policy.

The first local authority that employed welfare rights worker was in Oxfordshire County Council in 1969 (sadly the post was abolished in 1971 when the postholder left). This was followed by Manchester City Council in 1972 and others including Newcastle City Council in 1974. At this point, welfare rights 'teams' began to be created in several other local authorities and individual posts started to grow from just one or two posts into fully functioning units complete with administrative support (usually in councils' social services or social work departments). By the end of 1976 one study showed that between 25 and 30 local authorities employed at least one welfare rights officer (Fimister 1986: 47). In the late 1970s (through to the mid-1980s), government funded job creation schemes were a source of funding for welfare rights advice posts within both local authorities and the voluntary sector.

A landmark event occurred in April 1976 when Frank Field (then Director of CPAG and now a Member of Parliament associated with the harsher edges of modern social security policy) received a package containing leaked Cabinet minutes. These revealed that the then Labour government, newly led by Jim Callaghan, who had replaced Wilson as premier that month, was planning to abandon a manifesto pledge to introduce universal child benefit (something which had been a key CPAG policy since its formation). Field promptly passed on the leaked papers to the *Guardian* newspaper, which published it on the front page. Within six weeks the government was forced into a humiliating, public climbdown and child benefit was introduced (McCarthy 1986: 269).

No one now doubts that Frank Field did the right thing and it exposed a classic case of political sophistry at the heart of government which would have intensified poverty for millions of families in subsequent years. Even though by handling leaked secret papers he may have been technically breaking the law, it was a brave thing to do and is an example of the challenging and assertive tactics often necessary in the welfare rights field.

The election of Margaret Thatcher's government in 1979 and the decades which followed heralded an escalation in the need for welfare rights work and the development of welfare rights services; however, this was accompanied by a squeeze on the local authorities' ability to fund such work. As a government committed to implementing free market economic polices, curbing public spending (particularly welfare related expenditure), allowing less competitive businesses to fold and using unemployment as an economic tool to control inflation ('Unemployment is the price worth paying for lower inflation': Chancellor of the Exchequer, Norman Lamont), the inevitable result was the growth in inequalities and poverty which still characterises UK society today. Official unemployment (the measurement of which was 'adjusted' over 30 times, mostly to reduce the figures until 1997) rose from 1.07 million in May 1979 to 2.1 million in May 1985, continuing to rise to a peak of 3 million in May 1985 and staying above 2 million until November 1996, thence down to below 1 million in February 2001 (source: Office for National Statistics Seasonally Adjusted Claimant Count: www.nomis.co.uk).

There were other drivers for welfare rights advice – such as increased numbers of lone parents, recognition of groups who had been ignored such as carers and younger disabled people, retired people on fixed/low incomes who were brought into poverty by high inflation and the broken link between pensions and earnings. While unemployed people were never a major source of referrals for many welfare rights agencies, the consequential effect of government policies on benefits, taxation and unemployment increased advice needs among these groups.

During the 1980s a continuous process of paring back benefit entitlement took place. Early measures included the abolition of earnings related supplement to un-employment and sickness benefits, the restricting of supplementary benefit exceptional needs payments in 1980, reducing annual increases in long-term benefits to the inflation index for prices rather than earnings (which at the time of writing is estimated to have cumulatively reduced the real value of benefits by nearly 30 per cent) and the outright abolition of several non-means-tested benefits.

The combined effect of rising joblessness, increased low pay which accompanied the reduced demand for unskilled labour and the extension of means testing by stealth was that the number of people receiving supplementary benefit/income support rose from 566,000 in 1979 to over 2.94 million in just ten years – more than a fivefold increase. Of course this had the paradoxical effect for a government committed to reducing public expenditure, of increasing spending on benefits from £18.7 billion to £47.3 billion in cash terms. However, the effect of the successive cuts in benefits during this period is illustrated by the fact that despite the dramatic increase in benefit recipients, real expenditure on benefits rose only 25.8 per cent and as a proportion of gross domestic product only rose from 9.17 per cent to 9.84 per cent (source: Institute for Fiscal Studies Fiscal Facts www.ifs.org.uk).

Of course these figures fail to show the impact on other public services of this rising poverty and it was in this context that welfare rights activity and services experienced their greatest growth, particularly within local authorities. Such growth (as was the case for local authority anti-poverty strategies in general) took place in spite of the relentless squeeze on local government finance, reflecting the high priority that local authorities gave to such activity.

It was also during this era that organisations such as the National Campaign Against Social Security Cuts, a coalition of claimant activists, trade unions, local authorities and voluntary bodies, formed and campaigned for several years against the cuts and restrictions brought about by the government.

Also in 1981, Joan McClintock, then Director of the Australian Council of Social Service, visited the UK on a study tour and wrote a report the following year (McClintock 1982) recommending the establishment of welfare rights services based on the UK model across Australia. Within ten years all Australian states had developed and funded such services and there still exists a flourishing national body, the National Welfare Rights Network. Any welfare rights adviser in the UK would recognise the style and types of activity in Australia. However, in the recent past the Liberal/National Coalition government has

> actively sought to silence non-government advocacy groups . . . and has defunded a number of welfare advocacy groups and has sought to limit the access and influence of other interest groups . . . which receive government funding. For example, the Howard Government issued a statement in August 1999 requesting that funded bodies work collaboratively with the Department of Family and Community services . . . this request appeared to be designed to muzzle funded bodies by reducing them to agents of government.
>
> (Mendes 2004: 11–15)

Sadly it appears that little has developed in New Zealand, even in the face of the drastic cuts in benefit entitlement implemented by successive governments there.

COMING OF AGE – THE 1988 REFORMS AND BEYOND

The year 1988 heralded major reforms to the social security system in the UK with substantial cuts in and restructuring of housing benefit, the abolition of supplementary benefit and its replacement by income support which paid less to people under 25 and less to people with additional needs, further paring back of non-means-tested benefits and the introduction of the discretionary, non-appealable, and mostly loan-based Social Fund for one-off exceptional needs. The Social Fund proposals in particular galvanised opposition to these reforms because the government had originally proposed that local authority social workers and others would play a part in deciding who qualified for help. A broad coalition of opposition developed ranging from the Association of Directors of Social Services to the local authority associations and professional and trade union bodies. There were three main results from this activity and which were key in shaping welfare rights activity in the UK to this day.

First, it spurred local authorities to further invest in welfare rights services, primarily in-house services. By May 1986 research by the Policy Studies Institute showed that 30 per cent of all local authorities already had salaried welfare rights staff, rising to 61 per cent of the urban-based metropolitan councils. However, most had fewer than six staff and only 20 per cent had more than nine staff. In addition, at the time there were 1,236 generalist advice agencies outside local authorities providing welfare rights advice to some degree or another (Berthoud *et al.* 1986).

Second, welfare rights services and local authorities across the UK ran publicity campaigns (often with back-up help and advice) to encourage claimants to claim the additional help available under the old scheme before its provisions expired. An interesting initiative was undertaken by the then Scottish Strathclyde Council, promulgated by Welfare Rights Officer Chris Orr to get higher 'long-term' rates of supplementary benefit for long-term unemployed people in their fifties. Staff from several local authorities also established a national initiative with pre-printed claim materials in 1987 to 'Claim them before it's too late. They'll go in '88'. Such work was both a direct anti-poverty measure as well as a way of politicising the issue by showing up the stark contrast between the old and new systems and this activity was frequently not well received by DHSS officials, who responded by procrastinating and overzealously refusing claims (subsequently often won on appeal). The scale of activity in this period was so huge that I cannot begin to do justice to it.

Third, it enabled the local authority associations and others to effectively resist the involvement of local authority staff as partners in the widely unpopular benefits system and to affirm their role as advocates. The three main local authority associations, Convention of Scottish Local Authorities, Association of Metropolitan Authorities and Association of County Councils, issued a policy statement of 'Determined Advocacy' against the Social Fund.

For local authorities whose political controlling group was opposed to the Conservatives, developing such services made good political sense as well as a way of providing a practical response for the public. It was almost a badge of opposition to national government if your authority had a Women's Unit, a Race Equality Unit and Welfare Rights Unit – all three indicating that you were committed to protecting and promoting the rights of groups who were marginalised and disadvantaged by national policies. And while the former two services have become mainstream features of not just local government but most of the public and private sectors too, welfare rights services are often still a marginal service – an inevitable result of challenging benefit practices and advocating for socially unpopular groups and causes.

However, it was by no means the case that all such developments were within Opposition controlled local authorities. I started the welfare rights service in the then Conservative controlled Suffolk County Council in 1986 and in the same era Conservative controlled councils as diverse as Hereford and Worcestershire, Hertfordshire and Kent, all developed in-house welfare rights services which continue to this day, while many others increased spending on welfare rights services in external organisations. The debate was usually about use of the title 'Welfare Rights'. Some of this was driven by old-style, one-nation Conservatism, where concern for the deserving poor was still acceptable. On other occasions it was driven by self-interest, as welfare rights units increasingly demonstrated the economic case for increasing the income of people in impoverished areas – for example, giving them an increased ability to pay local authority taxes and charges, and the wider positive economic impact on economically disadvantaged communities from increased benefit take-up.

It is a sign of the times that having successfully and relatively easily persuaded senior managers and Conservative councillors in Suffolk, during the Thatcher era, to use the term 'Welfare Rights Unit', a decade of local New Labour rule resulted in the dropping of this title in favour of 'Financial Inclusion and Advice Service'. Similar name changes have occurred elsewhere.

Having become embedded within local authorities, it became increasingly clear that welfare rights services and activity (whether or not carried out by welfare rights specialists) had a key role to play in anti-poverty strategies and in also providing strategic advice and support on the relationships between social security and a range of local authority services – everything from clarifying entitlement to free school meals in local authority publicity to strategic advice about the benefit efficient design of residential care services.

The development of local authority anti-poverty strategies flowed very naturally from the increase in poverty taking place before the eyes of local authority officers and councillors and inevitably, they frequently looked to welfare rights staff for expertise and guidance about such strategies. Welfare rights work was and remains an effective and relatively cheap way to respond to poverty – indeed, it is hard to conceive of an effective and credible anti-poverty strategy which does not include benefit income maximisation as an activity. Work by the Association of Metropolitan Authorities in 1990 confirmed that not only had the number of local authorities with an anti-poverty strategy increased since the 1988 reforms but also many were closely linked to welfare rights services (Balloch and Jones 1990).

Anti-poverty strategies also represented a reaction to the prevailing tone of the Thatcher government, which was that poverty no longer existed. For example, in an early speech to the Conservative Political Centre on 11 May 1989, John Moore, then

Secretary of State for Social Services and responsible for implementing the 1988 social security reforms, stated that: 'poverty is a thing of the past . . . inequalities are an inevitable product of a increasingly affluent society'.

I can also well remember being asked on several occasions to remove the 'p' word from written reports to Conservative politicians because they would find this 'embarrassing'. On another occasion, suggesting at a meeting with government officials that one might see the Community Care reforms of 1992 as part of a wider movement to tackle poverty, I was firmly but politely told by the senior civil servant chair that: 'Ministers would find such a concept too philosophical'.

The Community Care reforms have their origins in government anxieties about the level and growth of social security spending on people in residential care homes. The system in place prior to 1993 meant that care homes had a perverse incentive to increase and maintain fees at the higher levels of supplementary benefit/income support then paid to people living in care homes. Expenditure had grown at a faster rate than other areas and there was an openly stated desire to cap this spending. The Griffiths Report of 1988, *Community Care: An Agenda for Action*, proposed the ending of this stream of finance and for placements to occur only after social work assessments by local authorities, which in turn would have benefits expenditure transferred to them in order to pay for care homes fees and/or to provide or arrange community based alternatives. Initially met with scepticism by Margaret Thatcher, the Community Care changes were implemented after a long period of planning by central and local government.

The relationship between social security rights and local government's finance needs became increasingly clear to local authorities, who frequently turned to welfare rights staff for strategic advice in devising benefit efficient models of care. The relationship between benefits and the care system was (and often remains) a particularly complex and obscure aspect of an already complicated and muddled web. As Fimister says:

> Social security as it relates to community care represents one of the most difficult aspects of a difficult system. If we look at benefit provisions overall, we can see that they are not only painfully complex, but also subject to a process of continuous change. At any given time, it is likely that one substantial upheaval or another is either under way or in the pipeline, or both; while batches of detailed amendment regulations arrive with alarming frequency . . . there is a certain macho 'complexity culture' pervading the drafting of benefit law. As an article in the Law Society Gazette put it (commenting on social security law in general but, but giving an example from the community care field): 'Cross-references – to sub-sections, to other sections, to schedules, to a myriad of regulations and indeed to other Acts proliferate. One finds exceptions to exceptions. Double and even triple negatives almost seem like a badge of honour: No self–respecting section is complete without one' . . . Or as Lord Justice Glidewell put it, in a case concerning the severe disability premium . . .' it is deplorable that legislation which affects some of the most disadvantaged people in society should be couched in language which is so difficult for even a lawyer trained and practising in this field to understand' (*Bate v Chief Adjudication Officer*,

Court of Appeal, 30.11.94) [[1996] 1 WLR 814]. For our present purposes,
suffice it to say that the grafting of the new community care arrangements
onto this system has created a good deal of bafflement on the ground as to
what benefits service users might be entitled to and what is the current state
of play as the rules of entitlement continue to mutate.

Nor, it might be added, is such bafflement only to be found at 'ground
level'. Senior civil servants in the relevant policy units and welfare rights
advisers working with the LA Associations have spent many long hours
arguing amongst themselves and with each other about what this or
that aspect of the law actually means, is intended to mean or achieves
in practice.

(Fimister 1995)

At a national level, experienced welfare rights staff played a key role in negotiations with government, protecting local authority and claimant interests by presenting
alterative options for changes to benefit rules, devising income maximisation strategies
(which would also benefit local authorities because of the revenue they could recoup
from service charges and/or by enabling people to live more independently, thus
reducing the need for services). The Community Care reforms were characterised
by what local authorities of all political control felt was shortfall in funding, so strategies
to maximise income became a priority. A detailed history of the changes, their
complexity and the role of welfare rights advisers is contained in Geoff Fimister's (1995)
book *Social Security and Community Care in the 1990s*.

Many local authorities increased their welfare rights provision as a result, steering
such services towards targeting users and potential users of community care services –
for example, in Hertfordshire, routinely screening people using the homecare service to
help them claim additional benefits. Alongside this, welfare rights services continued
the tradition of benefit take-up campaigns, some employing staff dedicated to running
benefit take-up initiatives. Particularly large-scale activity was undertaken by local
authorities such as Derbyshire County Council, Newcastle City Council and Manchester
City Council (by no means an exhaustive list), such activity being given added impetus
by the endless stream of changes to benefit rules. These changes were usually negative,
but the introduction of the disability living allowance in 1992 provided great scope
for raising awareness of this new benefit and also for addressing the shocking levels
of poverty among people with disabilities and long-term health needs. I doubt that the
Thatcher and John Major governments envisaged quite how far welfare rights advisers
would increase take-up of disability living allowance: this would become a cushion
against the severe cuts in benefits for this group implemented in 1988 and the growth
in health inequality caused by chronic poverty and joblessness – particularly in the
former industrial areas of the UK.

Disability living allowance has been a particularly fertile ground for test cases by
welfare rights advisers. The *Mallinson* case (an appeal started by Martin Rathfelder,
a Welfare Rights Officer with Manchester City Council, and which went all the way to
the House of Lords) radically extended its scope for people with sensory impairments.
Fairey/Halliday ensured that help with social activities could be counted towards

entitlement and *Moyna* has helped those with variable conditions. An uncountable number of cases appealed to the social security commissioners has also improved entitlement.

Test cases and the well-argued work of appeals up through the appellate process have also helped in all other areas of benefit entitlement and are a regular feature of work by welfare rights specialists.

The 1990s also saw the efforts to reshape social security customer services. This had mixed results – some DSS customer service staff were genuinely committed to improving services, others appeared to behave as if their priority was to protect the organisation. One side-effect was the outsourcing of work from London social security offices in an effort to improve services to claimants. This resulted in a spectacular failure of service to thousands of people, the problems being publicised and campaigned against by an organisation call Towerwatch (the name being taken from Euston Tower, one of the large London social security offices). This was a loose coalition of welfare rights advisers in local authorities and voluntary bodies, claimants and others. However, such examples of grass roots campaigns became increasingly unusual through the 1990s.

On the international front, the breakup of the Soviet bloc led to the establishment of Citizens Advice Bureaux in many eastern European countries – the advocacy involved in such activity would have been positively dangerous in the Soviet era. The first bureaux in Poland were set up in 1996, though there were none in Romania until 2002. In France legislation in 1999 compelled each department to establish a CASU (*Commission de l'action sociale d'urgence* – emergency social action commission). These act as advocates and brokers across welfare rights issues (including housing and training matters).

ACTIVITY 1.2

Identify the social, economic and political forces which drove the development of welfare rights activity and services.

NEW LABOUR – OLD FEARS

The election of Tony Blair's New Labour government in May 1997 created huge expectations for positive change in the benefits system. By this time it was estimated that 50 per cent of all local authorities had anti-poverty strategies, so political awareness of the issues which welfare rights advisers had been raising for decades had never been higher (Brown and Passmore 1998). It also appears that the number of local authorities (though not necessarily the number of staff) has doubled since the 1986 Policy Studies Institute survey (see Berthoud *et al.* 1986; Patterson 2001), meaning that 120 local authorities had some form of welfare rights service.

However, a pre-election public pledge by Blair and his Chancellor of the Exchequer, Gordon Brown, not to break the previous Conservative government's tax and spending polices meant that Labour was faced with implementing the Conservatives' previously planned benefit cuts – particularly cuts in appeal rights, cuts in benefits for lone parents alongside a new range of sanctions for benefit fraud and failure to comply with jobseeking activity.

Of great significance was the surprise announcement by Tony Blair in 2000 that his government aimed to abolish child poverty within twenty years. Freed from the shackles of the two-year tax and spending pledge, this eventually led, among other things, to a quiet and steady increase over the next few years in the family-related elements of means-tested benefits rates of over 80 per cent in real terms and a number of improvements in benefits for childcare, ultimately leading to the introduction of child tax credit in 2003.

Despite the initial fiscal caution, the Blair era has seen major reforms to the benefits system including the merger of jobsearch and benefits administrative functions of social security, a host of initiatives to address joblessness among young people, lone parents and those with a disability, major improvements to maternity benefits and the introduction of the tax credits scheme. On the debit side, we have seen the abolition of higher rates of benefit for new lone parents, the tightening of incapacity benefit entitlement ('the UK has some of the strictest eligibility criteria in the world' – DWP spokesman quoted in *Daily Mail*, 19 September 2004), serial restrictions on benefits for people from abroad (ostensibly to curb benefit tourism but without supporting evidence), the increasing use of benefit sanctions to compel people to adopt certain behaviour in order to receive benefits, the introduction by stealth of benefits with no right of appeal and the failure to resolve long-standing injustices such as Social Fund loans, restrictions on benefits for homeowners.

The major constitutional changes brought about by New Labour's decision to incorporate the European Convention on Human Rights into English, Scots and Northern Irish law in October 2000 via the Human Rights Acts have provided some long-term key principles previously lacking because of the UK's absence of a written constitution. In particular the Convention's provisions concerning rights to a fair trial (Article 6 of the Convention), rights to respect for private and family life (Article 8), prohibition of discrimination (Article 14) and protection of property (Article 1 of The First Protocol) give welfare rights advocates important additional arguments to protect the interests of claimants and to challenge the unfair basis of some legislation.

In parallel, means-tested benefits for older people have been gradually increased by record amounts. This was partly inspired by controversy about a 50 pence annual increase in state retirement pension in 2002. To avoid obvious presentational problems, the government has shied away from a formal public pledge to abolish pensioner poverty by a certain date, even though Gordon Brown was pressing his cabinet colleagues for a pledge about pensioner poverty from before the 2002 election. But low take-up of means-tested benefits by older people has remained a persistent problem, undermining the anti-poverty policy aims behind pension credit.

To stimulate the DWP into doing something, the Local Government Association launched a high profile national guide to benefit take-up for older people, *It's a Right . . . Not a Lottery* in 1998. The new ministerial team at the DWP was at least nominally committed to improving take-up, it having been included in the Labour Party's 1997 election manifesto and the idea having been taken up by the then shadow ministerial social security team at an informal meeting with local authority welfare rights advisers in 1995.

The DWP eventually launched a take-up campaign, initially choosing neither to work closely with local authorities nor to accept advice that was offered. The DWP's lack of experience and expertise in take-up work led to a poorly targeted but high profile publicity initiative which produced far worse returns on investment than those routinely achieved by local authorities. The Department for Work and Pensions has never publicly admitted the failings of its take-up strategy and *Income Take-up A Good Practice Guide* (Pension Service 2002) was edited by officials to tone down the presentation of findings which put the department in a poor light; the *Guide* received scant publicity, being published only after persistent lobbying by welfare rights interests.

The *Good Practice Guide* showed that:

- 77 per cent of all local authorities undertook some form of take-up work on income support and attendance allowance
- an estimated £57 million extra a year in benefits was awarded from this take-up work among the 46 per cent of local authorities who kept statistics
- 79 per cent of Citizens Advice Bureaux did take-up work with older people, though statistics on awards were less precise
- at the time, just 49 (8.9 per cent of the total) of local DWP offices undertook take-up work.

Difficulties with take-up led to the establishment of the national DWP and external agency Partnerships Against Poverty group and the first ever secondment (myself) from local government to advise on benefit take-up by older people in 2001. Products of this era included the toned down *Good Practice Guide* and various information leaflets.

Currently take-up of pension credit remains low at about 60 per cent (about the same level that income support take-up by older people reached), despite millions of pounds spent promoting it (£15.58 million in 2003 alone – Parliamentary Question 13 May 2004). The high profile publicity campaign also had the effect of encouraging 2.64 million people to ring the national Pension Credit Application Line in the first eight months of 2004, but only 30 per cent went on either to request a claim form or to make an application over the phone (Parliamentary Question /04/188683). Such a level of performance begs questions about the ability of the DWP to undertake effective benefit take-up initiatives. Data from voluntary and local authority welfare rights services show a distinct trend of far better performance and value for money, perhaps indicating higher levels of trust by older people and these services' ability to identify underclaimers.

New Labour's collective inferiority complex caused by years of painful internal strife and electoral rejection meant that they had become (and remain) intolerant of external criticism. At one meeting in 2000, Alastair Darling (then Secretary of State for Social Security) asked Sir Jeremy Beecham (then Chairman of the Local Government Association) to bear down on welfare rights activists who kept criticising the government and who 'seem to see themselves as some kind of advocates for the "oppressed"'.

Sir Jeremy, a wise man with firm principles, ignored this bizarre (and impractical) request. On another occasion in 2001, ministers were advised in writing by civil servants not to invite external partner organisations to the launch of a leaflet to increase benefit take-up by pensioners, because this might give such organisations an opportunity to criticise government policy.

Another landmark has been New Labour's uneasy relationship with disability benefits and the groups which represent the interests of those receiving these. Widespread unhappiness with the 1998 legislation which further tightened incapacity benefit entitlement was generally felt to have terminated the promising career of the then Secretary of State for Social Security, Harriet Harman. However, the increasingly open and personal conflicts between her and her deputy minister, Frank Field, which were acting as a block to effective reform, may have been as much of a factor in her subsequent exile from the cabinet. Internally New Labour has been concerned about figures which suggest an exponential growth in disability benefit expenditure. The figures are of course capable of interpretation in several ways and it is hard to assess how far civil service attitudes from a long period of Conservative rule were responsible for promoting the inaccurate view that disability benefits spending was out of control, but in 1997 onwards various disability organisations publicly campaigned against cuts in disability benefits. This culminated in two particularly public embarrassments: the self-chaining of disabled people to the gates of Downing Street with gallons of red paint thrown on the road and the walkout from consultation meetings by national disability groups. This led various ministers to view disability groups as an internal opposition. For example, it was widely believed within the then Department of Social Security that Secretary of State Alastair Darling did not want his staff meeting disability organisations on his department's premises and only after he had agreed to any such meetings.

Social work and welfare rights interests became associated with the disability lobby because of the great significance of disability benefits to their customers. Although the representative bodies such as the Local Government Association and Association of Directors of Social Services adopted a less confrontational approach, they sought to influence government policy so that further cuts were not taken forward. Welfare rights staff in local authorities and voluntary organisations were involved in such lobbying as well as providing expert technical help – perhaps further adding to New Labour distrust of the welfare rights perspective on matters and the off-the-cuff comment to Sir Jeremy Beecham to clamp down on welfare rights services.

It was also during this period that pension credit found its way onto the statute books. Officially called State Pension Credit, government lawyers advised against the use of the term 'pension credit' because of the existence of another similarly worded concept elsewhere in social security law, so Gordon Brown and Alastair Darling, despite advice from officials about the negative connotations of the word 'credit' in the eyes of many pensioners, simply put the word 'state' in front to officially name this new benefit. Paradoxically, despite the desire that this benefit should be simple, it has proved to be extremely complex to explain to lay people and the near impossibility of precisely predicting who does or does not qualify has undoubtedly contributed to a laggardly take-up rate.

Also victims of New Labour's politics are local authority anti-poverty strategies. While many local authorities have mainstreamed most or some of such strategies into their corporate planning processes, many in the welfare rights field have observed that numerous local authorities have also discarded them or toned them down and renamed them 'Social Inclusion Strategies'. The paradox is of a government committed to ending poverty among key groups, while local authorities downgrade their anti-poverty work. Government has not helped by frequently making its anti-poverty pledges in a whisper for fear of alienating its more rightwing supporters.

A further challenge is posed by the increasingly close organisational links between local authorities and the DWP – ostensibly in the name of social inclusion and joined up governance, but weakening the ability of local authority councillors and staff to act as advocates for their communities and customers.

In the New Labour era some welfare rights provision has benefited from a number of areas of government policy and growing expenditure – benefits advice delivered in health settings has been a growth area as part of wider action by the National Health Service and local authorities to reduce health inequalities, the Sure Start projects have funded some welfare rights advice as has community regeneration activity and in England and Wales there is now substantial funding from the Legal Services Commission (albeit with significant strings attached to the funding).

Among non-welfare rights specialists, the perception is that social workers have gradually retreated from involvement in welfare rights advice and advocacy as local authorities focus on the specific targets and service priorities government has decreed for them. This is despite the inclusion of benefits check as part of several government driven reforms to social care services (such as the Fairer Charging guidance and the National Service Framework for Children). Within social housing there has been a noticeable growing engagement of staff in welfare rights work – partly inspired by external pressure by various inspectorate bodies and the realisation that welfare rights work helps reduce rent arrears but also because housing providers increasingly see themselves as providers of broader services than just bricks and mortar.

Today, despite current challenges, welfare rights practice remains a key feature of the work of many people employed in the public sector, be they welfare rights specialists or not. The external policy agenda has altered but the activity has remained essentially the same across national borders and through changes in benefit entitlement – advocating on behalf of people entitled to benefits to maximise their entitlement. Much of our welfare rights practice nowadays remains essentially the same as when I started in the early 1970s – rather like the same music but played by a different band. Despite new benefits, new technology and the discovery of customer care by benefits administrators, it frequently revolves around challenging bad benefit decisions caused by poor training, indecipherable legislation and unacceptable attitudes, helping people claim who have had obvious entitlement for years and who were never helped to claim by benefit administrators, chasing up constant delays and administrative failures by benefit providers, pushing back the boundaries of entitlement through test cases and lobbying for improvements. To quote a cliché: *plus ça change, plus c'est la même chose* (the more things change, the more they remain the same).

This chapter has put welfare rights practice into a historical, international and philosophical context. Chapter 2 examines the scope and nature of welfare rights work in everyday practice, the current and future policy climate and further examines the ethical basis for effective welfare rights activity.

MODERN WELFARE RIGHTS PRACTICE

OBJECTIVES

By the end of this chapter you should:

▪ Understand the political, economic and social forces which shape welfare rights work

▪ Recognise the implications of these for practice

▪ Be able to clarify the links between poverty and ill health and how welfare rights practice can help reduce health inequalities

▪ Understand how welfare rights practice fits with social work practice

▪ Understand the impact of the modern public service management culture.

THE CURRENT ENVIRONMENT FOR WELFARE RIGHTS PRACTICE

Welfare rights practice is now a mature activity and while it may not always be welcomed by politicians in power, it is an activity which will not cease: the forces which create the environment for it are just too strong and it would continue even if all welfare rights organisations ceased to exist and if all their books were burned.

The need for welfare rights activity nowadays is as great as it has ever been – if not more so than when it started in the 1960s. The pressures which create a need for welfare rights work (not in any particular order) are discussed in this chapter and these are as follows:

- Ever more means testing
- Who's on the fiddle? The anti-fraud drive
- Actually, they get it wrong
- Work is the best form of welfare
- The grand pledge: abolishing child and pensioner poverty
- Not welcome here: migration and social security law
- Always with us: the persistence of serious levels of poverty and inequality
- Growing by the day: increasing numbers of older people
- Some die sooner: health inequalities
- A safe home? Welfare rights and housing
- Welfare rights practice by social workers
- We're all managers now.

EVER-MORE MEANS TESTING

There is a neverending growth of means testing in the social security system. Not only have successive governments since 1979 almost continually trimmed non-means-tested benefits (a process which pushes more people below means-tested benefits thresholds as their income falls relative to those thresholds), but also new benefits have been developed which encompass wider sections of the population. In recent years two key developments in social security have been the implementation of pension credit for people aged 60 or older and tax credits, several elements of which are aimed at people in work. With 85 per cent of UK families having a potential entitlement to child tax credit, means testing on an almost universal scale is now an entrenched policy.

The position of benefits for older people also illustrates the growth of means testing. The number of older people entitled to pension credit is estimated to be 4.65 million in 2005–06, growing to a staggering 6.35 million by 2014–15; each year over 100,000 more older people become entitled (Parliamentary Questions 23 July 2004). This is of course in addition to the approximately 20 per cent annual pension credit caseload turnover mainly because of death rates.

A primary cause of the additional number of people who are entitled is the fact that retirement pension increases in line only with prices whereas part of pension credit increases in line with earnings. When the first forerunner of pension credit, supplementary pension, was introduced in 1965 as a safety net for poorer pensioners who did not have adequate retirement provision, it would have been political suicide for politicians to even jokingly suggest that the majority of older people should be eligible for a means-tested benefit.

The problems associated with means testing are well illustrated by problems with pension credit. With a government target of getting just 73 per cent of eligible pensioners (6 million) to receive this benefit by 2006, take-up is a challenge and it is possible that even this modest target will not be achieved, and all the assumptions about the redistributive effects of pension credit assume 100 per cent take-up rates. If such a rate was achieved, the poorest decile of pensioners would gain an average additional income of 8.1 per cent compared to 0.3 per cent among the richest decile (Brewer and Emmerson 2003: 7). But persistently low take-up rates would 'seriously limit the government's ability to help lower income pensioners' (Brewer and Emmerson 2003: 8) and may actually make inequality among this group worse.

Means testing as a vehicle for delivering benefits has significant drawbacks which all create a need for welfare rights work – whether by specialists or non-specialists. Here are some reasons why:

- Means-tested benefits never achieve full take-up levels – one is forever coming across people who have missed out.
- Customers of the benefits system need more help and support claiming them – sometimes time spent filling in a claim form is time well invested if it saves more serious problems later on.
- Inevitably, the legislation is dense and complicated – particularly for those who are unfamiliar with the system.
- It creates a great likelihood of delay, error, overpayment and administrative failure. A huge amount of time is spent by claimants and their advisers trying to manage and challenge such problems.
- The intricate rules of entitlement create enormous potential for disputes and challenge – the rules can be read in various ways. The trick in welfare rights practice is to apply the most favourable interpretation.
- They are time consuming and demoralising for benefits officials to administer, thus increasing staff turnover and weakening the pool of collective knowledge
- They create poverty traps which in turn create disincentives to take on paid work.
- The UK's interrelated system of means-tested benefits with passported entitlements is like a chain – it is only as strong as the weakest link and any single link can fail.

Resolving problems with or even calculating means-tested benefits (particularly for service users with multiple means-tested benefits and tax credit entitlement) can be complex, time-consuming and frustrating and are sometimes put forward as a rationale for welfare rights work to be done only by 'experts'. While the complexity and impenetrability of present-day multiple benefit means testing makes life difficult even for advisers with good computer benefits calculation software, it does not logically mean that involvement in welfare rights practice is an all or nothing option and there is still plenty of scope for involvement by non-experts.

There are few signs that the government's addiction to means testing as a vehicle for social security delivery is at the point where they recognise the need to reduce dependence, let alone take steps towards abstinence. But it is possible that adjustments will be made in the long-term to benefits for older people in order to reduce the extent of means testing (and also to perhaps save some political face) and many still live in hope that child benefit will be increased sufficiently so that less people have to rely on means-tested benefits. But whichever party is in government, means testing will continue to be responsible for a major part of our benefits system and to continue to produce bucket loads of work for advisers. Even if non-means-tested benefits were radically reformed so that they largely replaced means-tested benefits, one would still need an element of means-tested provision in order to provide cover for those who do not qualify for non-means-tested benefits.

WHO'S ON THE FIDDLE? THE ANTI-FRAUD DRIVE

The pursuit of benefit claimants alleged to be receiving benefits dishonestly has been a continual theme in social policy since the 1980s. Each of the major parties tries to outdo the other in claims of effectiveness about their clampdown on benefit fraud – rather like they used to with housebuilding pledges in the 1960s.

While there always has been benefits fraud (just as there has always been a bigger problem with tax evasion by wealthier people) many of the claims about the scale of benefit fraud are highly questionable. For example, the DWP's routinely issued figures for 'Fraud and Official Error' include all manner of estimated overpayments, by no means all fraudulent, and also include figures for cases where the DWP has made a mistake and overpaid the claimant.

Local authority figures for the level of fraud are even more incredible. Each local authority is required to keep 'weekly benefit savings' figures. These show that, for example, in 2000–01 local authorities detected £133.9 million in housing and council tax benefit fraud, yet the DWP which administers vastly greater amounts of benefit uncovered just £16.38 million (Parliamentary Question 151019 12 March 2004). The DWP's Benefit Fraud Inspectorate has also regularly criticised local authorities for producing Weekly Benefit Savings Figures which are not supported by reliable evidence.

> The political imperative of headline figures and demand for success stories stifle the opportunity for a more imaginative examination of the fraud figures and for putting fraud in any form of external perspective. For example, in the public debates about fraud, why are the following never mentioned?
>
> • Social security fraud is only a fraction of the size of the informal economy, estimated by Lord Grabiner in a report published in 2000 to be worth between £50 billion and £80 billion.
> • Much of the money 'lost' to the social security system through fraud and error can be recovered from claimants. The statistics on the amounts recovered are not made public however.
> • The level of unclaimed income-related benefits is comparable to levels of fraud. In 1997–98 between £1.6 billion and £4.1 billion was not claimed.
>
> Our understanding of fraud is getting better, but the standard of public debate is not keeping pace.
>
> (Sainsbury 2001)

Every welfare rights adviser has examples of fraud cases where the amounts alleged to have been overpaid turn out to be inflated, not legally recoverable or when offset against unclaimed benefits and tax credits turn out to be de minimus amounts. We also each have our example of heavy handedness by fraud investigators. Personally, over the years I have dealt with cases where claimants credibly complained about threats to deport boyfriends, inappropriate questions about people's sexual activities, sexual harassment by fraud staff, intimidating interviews and negative racial stereotyping. While most fraud staff are probably as professional as any other benefits administrators and while the government has taken steps to tackle poor practice, it is of concern that such examples can be so readily cited.

While many fraud allegations turn out to be unfounded (witness the annual ratio of over a million calls to various fraud hotlines and the few hundred resulting prosecutions) and there can be much to advocate about to protect claimants from excessive behaviour and to challenge claims that they have received too much public money, the experience of a fraud investigation can traumatise individual claimants and creates a climate of paranoia which undermines efforts by all public officials to develop accessible, customer-focused public services.

On a wider level, the continued emphasis on fraud deters many people from claiming what they are legitimately entitled to (amounting to a mixed message when combined with government efforts to improve benefit take-up by certain groups), adds to prejudices about certain socially unpopular groups (such as young single parents) and creates a political climate which makes it easy to argue for cuts in benefits and against improvements. Welfare rights advisers in other countries report similar experiences.

Public debate on benefit fraud is rarely inconvenienced by close attention to facts. For example, most asylum seekers have been denied access to benefits since 1996 and they receive payments at 80 per cent of the very basic benefit rates via a bureaucratic and almost discretionary alternative system. Yet public perception is that asylum seekers live a life of luxury and have more favourable treatment than the general population. This unchecked and inaccurate perception then undermines both community relations and welfare benefit take-up, by associating claiming with being an undeserving scrounger.

It is likely that the anti-fraud agenda will continue in its current shape for years to come. It creates an additional dimension and need for people to be engaged in welfare rights practice.

ACTUALLY, THEY GET IT WRONG

A huge amount of welfare rights practice is concerned with correcting mistakes of benefit bureaucracies. The scale and type of errors which arise are never ending (and never cease to amaze) and one of the most frustrating aspects of welfare rights practice is knowing that you are right when the other side obstinately insists that they are right when they have plainly got matters upside down. This problem is amplified by the senior management culture of denial which pervades so much of the DWP, local authorities and HM Revenue and Customs.

The scale of error making by the DWP in particular is at least available publicly (one wishes that local authority housing benefit services were so transparent). In 2005 the DWP Decision Making Standards Committee's Report showed how widespread is just the admitted and measurable scale of basic errors in social security decision making, for example:

• failing to award the severe disability premium in income support amounting to underpayments of £257 million in the previous five years
• getting the National Insurance contribution rules for incapacity benefit wrong – an underpayment of £239 million
• misunderstanding rules about how incapacity benefit claims are linked – underpayments of £192 million
• not actioning incapacity benefit claim forms.

Even the more customer-focused Pension Service does not escape comment. Referring to the scale of mistakes in pension credit assessments, the committee comments that because things were so bad 'there was managerial checking of 100 per cent workloads for periods. This is likely to have the effect of producing more accurate results than would be the norm'. Despite such close supervision, missing the additional payments for pensioners with a severe disability 'results in high underpayments for the most vulnerable pensioners'.

On the disability benefits front, confirmation is given for what every advice worker has experienced – the appalling number of disability living allowance appeals which are refused and then defended at appeal by the DWP, despite strong evidence of entitlement.

Depressingly, it is stated that: 'It is not clear that the Department gives high priority to the quality of decision making' (Department for Work and Pensions Decision Making Standards Committee 2005).

The appallingly bad levels of decision making mean that there is likely to be a long-term and huge need for an independent source of advice simply to check and challenge such things. We all long for the day when we could focus on unavoidable and genuine disputes about entitlement. The reality is that such a day is a long way off.

WORK IS THE BEST FORM OF WELFARE

One of the successes of the Blair government has been to continually reduce joblessness and to introduce a range of reforms to make the tax and benefits system better at supporting people who move into paid work from benefits as their main source of income. Measures such as disability discrimination legislation, investment in skills training and the national minimum wage have also been key complementary elements in this strategy. Between 1997 and 2004, the number claiming benefits because of unemployment fell by over 2 million and other measures of joblessness also showed similar falls. However, there is evidence of workless people disappearing off the unemployment count because of long-term sickness. This is unsurprising given the considerable evidence of the damage that long-term unemployment does to one's health – even after standardising the data for age, 19.1 per cent of long-term unemployed men have a health problem compared to 8.5 per cent of men in unskilled manual work and 4.2 per cent of men who are managers or professionals (Babb *et al.* 2004: 76). Many advice workers have also noticed a growing phenomenon of young unemployed men who, humiliated by the process of claiming and the ever-present threat of benefit sanctions or because of cultural expectations, simply refuse to register as unemployed and claim benefits and who instead finance themselves through informal and/or illegal economic activity. Case-based research suggests a small but significant number of self-employed people in the informal economy who have opted out of legitimising their status in order to survive economically (Copisarow and Barbour 2004). Further corroboration is found in the fact that only between 55 and 70 per cent of those entitled to Jobseeker's Allowance actually claim it (DWP 2004a).

Official statistics also suggest some additional support for the existence of this phenomenon. The gap between the International Labour Office (ILO) and the Claimant Count methods of measuring unemployment has grown in recent years with approximately 550,000 unemployed people who are not 'signing on' with the DWP as unemployed (P. Bivand, personal communication, 2004). While some of this may be partly explained by the way that the ILO measure is done (e.g. people in full-time education who are looking for work appear in the ILO count), as well as highlighting the need for more research into this topic, it also indicates that welfare rights work with unemployed people is a neglected area for welfare rights advisers, who have had to become tied to local authority and health service priorities and the groups (such as children and pensioners) these bodies prioritise.

However, for other groups, the introduction of tax credits and other benefits to better support people in work means that

> the government's work-based welfare policy now delivers £6.5 billion of *extra* money to British families each year, compared to the annual rate of subsidy in 1997. More families now work and even the out-of-work families are £40 a week better off in real terms.
>
> (Marsh and Vegeris 2004, original emphasis)

But New Labour takes matters further by setting a target for an 80 per cent employment rate among the working age population (the rate in 2004 was 74.7 per cent) and seeing work per se as a solution: 'A job is the best route out of poverty' (Johnson 2004). But this fails to recognise the insecure and unsatisfactory nature of many of the jobs on offer to benefit claimants, who may also be compelled by threats from benefit officials to cut their benefits, into taking such work. Support for this view is offered from academic research:

> While work strongly reduces the risk of being in poverty, it does not eliminate it: two fifths of people in low-income working-age households

now have someone in paid work. Around seven million workers earn less than £6.50 an hour . . . low pay is only one of the disadvantages of jobs at the bottom of the labour market. In terms of job security, two fifths of people who find work no longer have that work six months later, the same proportion as a decade ago.

(New Policy Institute and Joseph Rowntree Foundation 2004: 4)

In addition, as the previous discussion about means testing highlights, the anti-poverty measures have predominantly taken place within the parameters of a profound commitment to retaining means testing as a major feature of our social security system with all the problems that this creates. Not the least of this is the increased difficulties for politicians caused by continuing to levy National Insurance contributions when such benefits are a diminishing feature of income maintenance which 'reinforces the perception that National Insurance Contributions are personal taxes by another name' (Social Security Advisory Committee 2004a: v).

The extract from one of Blair's speeches where he stated, 'Work for those who can, Security for those who cannot', is ostensibly the principle behind the New Labour welfare reforms. However, much of the benefits system is a very insecure place for many of the recipients with a failure to address basic weaknesses such as low levels of benefits for many claimants and the widespread existence of state sponsored debt through the loans element of the Social Fund.

> Labour's difficulties of engaging with what 'real' security might involve for those who cannot work are tied up with its confusion between those who 'cannot' work (because of illness, disability, caring responsibilities and so on) and its belief that everyone on theory *can* and *should* work. There is a sense that Labour equates those who cannot work with another group of workless people – those who *won't* work.
>
> (Becker 2002: 17)

This view was later illustrated by the unevidenced statement by DWP Minister Jane Kennedy in a speech to a Social Market Foundation seminar in December 2004 that: 'a third of the [incapacity benefit] claimants could work immediately and another third in the longer term' (*Guardian* 15 December 2004). I have been informally advised that the minister made 'a mistake' but the DWP does not appear to have tried to correct this public and damaging error and it was on the back of such statements that the DWP's five year plan in 2005 (DWP 2005) heralded the major changes in incapacity benefit which involve additional work-seeking expectations, greater use of DWP staff discretion (in view of past form, this is a worrying thing) and potential major cuts in the living standards of sick and disabled people (Reith 2005: 2). The DWP's planning assumption is that a million people will move off incapacity benefit and into work. This seems far fetched given that, at the time of writing, there are fewer than 700,000 vacancies nationally (many of which require skills and experience not generally found among incapacity benefit claimants) and the poor health of so many on incapacity benefit means that they are unlikely to be attractive candidates to most employers.

Already, the political pressure to get sick people into jobs produces an endless stream of appeals about people's ability and inability to work and the extent of their disability, with frequent noises from senior politicians about the alleged need to crack down on those 'languishing' on benefits for disability or ill health. Despite such rhetoric, the poor quality of decisions by benefit administrators to refuse benefits is illustrated by the fact that consistently, well over half of all claimants who are refused, and who appeal with representation, succeed in having benefits awarded or restored. Protecting and advocating for people claiming these benefits (and the proposed replacements in from 2008) is likely to remain a key feature of welfare rights work for many years to come.

Government policy on benefits for the long-term sick is frequently reactive and appears to be driven by prejudice. Despite the official line that 'The capability assessments for incapacity claimants are among the toughest in the world' (DWP spokesman quoted in *Daily Mail* 19 August 2004), by conceding the case for cuts in entitlement, the government gives credibility to ill-informed and hysterical criticisms such as: 'not a scintilla of reform has been achieved . . . the system is clearly failing. It is a huge burden on the taxpayer. And it encourages the hopeless, debilitating, soul destroying culture of handouts and lies' (*Daily Mail* editorial 19 August 2004).

A further very real problem with the New Labour welfare reform agenda, and its umbilical-like adherence to means testing, lies in the disincentives that means testing creates because of the poverty trap effect when benefits are withdrawn as income rises (see Figure 2.1).

Assuming there are no administrative failures when moving into work and also that someone knows of and succeeds in claiming their maximum entitlement,

> There are concerns that the Government's recent policy towards tax credits, of increasing the Child Tax Credit for the poorer half of parents and eroding the value of the Working Tax Credit by freezing the point at which higher incomes reduce tax credit entitlements, may be unsustainable in the medium term because of its negative impact on work incentives . . . the unambiguously negative impact of Housing Benefit and Council Tax Benefit on work incentives remains one of biggest challenges to any government wanting to make work pay.
>
> (Brewer and Shephard 2004)

Another report from the same publisher and published on the same day highlighted that:

> The government's anti-poverty strategy has so far emphasised the importance of reducing the number of households, especially those with children, where nobody works. However, crossing the divide from 'welfare' into work is only part of the picture.
>
> It is now time to think more widely about people's welfare, both inside and outside work. Millions of people in low-paid, insecure jobs need better training and working conditions and incentives, in order to realise their full potential and improve their living standards.
>
> (Hirsch and Millar 2004)

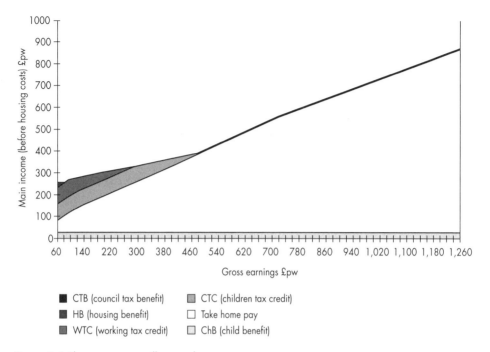

Figure 2.1 The poverty trap illustrated
Married couple with two children under 11, typical local authority tenant

Source: Department for Work and Pensions (2004) *Tax Benefit Model Tables.* Leeds: DWP

The graph shows the effect on take-home income when a family (DWP wording refers to a married couple) with an average local authority rent moves into full-time paid work. An allowance is built into the benefit level for passported benefits. It is not until about £450 a week gross is earned that this family start to see a good return on their income. The graph profiles preceding the introduction of tax credits showed a much flatter line (i.e. a worse poverty trap) and under the Conservatives, the line showed a declining real income at lower pay levels.

The ongoing changes to benefits and tax credits have produced and will continue to produce much work for welfare rights practitioners – unravelling the obscure complexities of tax credits, challenging tax credit over- and underpayments, advising claimants how to cope with dealing with up to eight different benefit and tax credit offices (many of whom appear to have chronic basic administrative deficiencies) and how to coordinate and manage the resulting interrelationships between the various payments they are responsible for. The complexity, which results from this massive extension of means testing, is clearly a barrier to involvement in welfare rights work by non-specialists. In addition, HM Revenue and Customs, which administers tax credits, appears to have a very different attitude towards claimants and their advisers compared to the DWP.

The matrix of different administrative mechanisms amplifies the inherent chain-like weaknesses in means-tested benefits and has undoubtedly made for an increased level of the type of welfare rights activity which involves basic progress chasing and doing better-off calculations for customers.

An interesting reflection on the changes is that: 'the term social security has virtually been removed from the lexicon' (Social Security Advisory Committee 2004a: iv).

A parallel development in the work and welfare world has been the introduction and gradual extension of 'work-focused' interviews and activities for all manner of benefit claimants (even though internal DWP research shows only a limited positive effect from such activities). Some of these have also been accompanied by undesirable and potentially discriminatory compulsion measures which either do not have rights of appeal or have only limited rights and which are clearly an exercise in social engineering through the social security system. There has also been a growth in discretionary measures with no formal rights of appeal.

The welfare to work policy agenda (particularly at a time of favourable economic circumstances) can easily hide the existence of widespread poverty:

> it must not be allowed to obscure the fact that there will always be a significant number of individuals who will never be able to sustain paid work – or in some cases any form of work at all.
>
> (Social Security Advisory Committee 2004a: iv)

The same advisory body also goes on to question the role of benefits administrators in moving people into work:

> the extent to which it is appropriate for Personal Advisers, with the control of benefits and the threat of sanction, actually to lead this process is questionable. So too is the [DWP's] capacity to recruit, train and indeed afford, individuals of the calibre needed for this work.
>
> (Social Security Advisory Committee 2004: iv)

ACTIVITY 2.1

Identify cases you are aware of when the benefits system has undermined people's efforts to enter or re-enter paid or unpaid work.

THE GRAND PLEDGE: ABOLISHING CHILD AND PENSIONER POVERTY

In contrast to Ireland, where successive governments have worked to implement a holistic anti-poverty strategy since 1986, the Blair government has limited its most public anti-poverty measures to two of the 'deserving' groups: children and older people. One effect has been to create a two-tier income maintenance system with benefit levels for single unemployed and childless people who are long-term sick remaining at scandalously low levels – dubbed by the *Guardian* newspaper in 2004 as 'The forgotten corner of the welfare state'.

All of the fall in the number of people in low-income households has been among children (and their parents) and pensioners. In 2002/03, 3.6 million children were in low-income households compared with 4.3 million in 1996/97, a fall of 700,000. 2.2 million pensioners were in low-income households compared with 2.7 million in 1996/97, a fall of 500,000. Pensioners are now no more likely to be in low-income than working-age households.

. . . In contrast, the number of working-age adults without dependent children in low income was higher in 2002/03 than in 1996/97: 3.9 million compared with 3.6 million. This group now accounts for a third of all people in low-income households.

The focus of Government anti-poverty strategies of recent years on children and pensioners, and the lack of priority accorded to working-age adults without dependent children, is illustrated by what has been happening to levels of Income Support (IS). Since 1998, IS for a couple with two children has risen by a third after allowing for inflation while IS for a couple with one child has risen a quarter. This rate of increase is greater than that for average earnings, which have risen by a sixth over the same period. By contrast, IS for working-age adults with no children has stayed unchanged (after allowing for inflation) over the whole ten-year period, falling ever further behind average incomes.

(New Policy Institute and Joseph Rowntree
Foundation 2004: 3)

However, the new and improved benefits for older people and carers of children which have followed in the wake of the pledges have created huge opportunities for welfare rights practitioners to identify people who are entitled. Benefit take-up work has been undertaken and aimed at these groups – for example, the high profile *Quids for Kids* initiative by the Local Government Association which started in 2003 (including highlighting examples of best practice around benefit take-up for families with disabled children) and numerous locally-based initiatives aimed at pensioners. These publications showcased examples of the huge amount of benefits take-up work with older people, those with disabilities and families with children and which has been going on well before any idea of benefit take-up became a glint in DWP officials' eyes in the late 1990s. Frustratingly, the contributions of both local authorities and voluntary organisations have received scant recognition by a DWP now allegedly committed to improving benefit take-up among some groups.

The scale of change in information and communication technology has opened up exciting new opportunities to identify underclaimers and to target them for help and advice. For example, work done routinely in Newcastle by the City Council's Welfare Rights Service using computerised housing benefit records to identify people who are missing out on other means-tested benefits has produced consistently strong results. Use of data warehouse technology by the London Borough of Newham to identify local residents who are underclaiming has produced (in 2003) a 31 per cent success rate gaining an average of £23.08 a week per person in additional benefits

(London Borough of Newham Social Regeneration Unit 2004) and 44 per cent success rate for working families tax credit claims among non-pensioners (Spence 2001).

Using a previous measure of poverty, the UK government reduced the number of children in poverty by 500,000 between 1998–99 and 2002–03 though various analysts have predicted that unless substantial improvements are made to benefits and taxation, the government may not hit its target to abolish child poverty by 2020 – even with changes to the measurement of poverty introduced in 2004 (Brewer *et al.* 2004). The poorest pensioners have seen their incomes rise by an average of £600 a year and this has brought about substantial reductions in absolute poverty for this group (DWP 2004b: 157). However, the government's target of getting only 70 per cent of older people who are eligible to actually receive pension credit means that the full anti-poverty effect will not be seen; the whole anti-poverty effect of this benefit relies on near 100 per cent take-up levels, which is unlikely given that take-up of means-tested benefits for older people has historically been at about 74 per cent. If it falls short, poverty remains a problem for many older people. To make for a greater challenge, take-up rates of council tax benefit among older people have actually fallen in recent years.

Later figures show a general continuation of these trends, hedged with some cautionary messages. For example, analysis by the Institute for Fiscal Studies shows that by 2003–04, child poverty had fallen by 100,000 to 3.5 million after housing costs (unchanged before housing costs are taken into account), and that

> to meet the government's short-term target, the number of children in poverty will now have to fall by 300,00 before housing costs and 500,000 after housing costs in 2004/05. The former still looks likely to be achieved, but the latter does not.
>
> (Brewer *et al.* 2005)

Much of the slow decline in child poverty was attributed by the authors to administrative problems with tax credits (a growing area of welfare rights practice). They also highlight that 'pensioner poverty continues to fall dramatically when incomes are measured after housing costs'.

Despite the progress, poverty levels in 2004–05 remained substantially higher than those of the 1970s and much work will be required over a very long period to address poverty among not only families with children and older people, but other groups as well. Welfare rights practice has to be a key component of such work.

The government has also become more committed to improving benefit take-up by pensioners and families with children – a significant contrast to the antipathy and ambiguity shown by previous governments. On the pensioner front, we have seen the deployment of local teams of DWP Pension Service staff to encourage take-up. Some of their efforts (such as outreach surgeries in public locations) have had very limited success and it is a pity that senior managers in the service did not accept the advice from welfare rights experts that such events produce few returns for the investment that this kind of activity involves. As mentioned earlier, there has also been significant national advertising and promotion of pension credit.

Benefit take-up can directly contribute to reductions in poverty. For example,

> data from the European Union show that cash benefits have an enormous impact on the poverty rate. In 1999 19 per cent of UK citizens were living in poverty: without benefits that figure would be 42 per cent. In Europe as a whole income poverty is at 15 per cent, which would rise to 40 per cent without benefits.
>
> (Jackson and Segal 2004: 50, citing
> Dennis and Guio 2003)

It is therefore a logical conclusion that increased benefit take-up by those on low incomes has positive effect on poverty levels. While welfare rights work may not always be central in this process, it certainly adds value and reaches people who would not otherwise make successful benefit claims. There is also evidence of the spending multiplier effect of benefit take-up in local communities, thus lending weight to the view that welfare rights work is also a useful part of economic regeneration activity. One tested economic model suggested that benefit take-up work in a low income London borough produced over £18 in the local economy for each £10 in additional benefit which is raised (Sacks 2002). Other research by economists at Strathclyde University concluded that the £10.795 million gained for people by Glasgow City Council's Welfare Rights Service in 2002–03 produced an additional 258 jobs (mostly long-term) across Scotland because of the additional spending power this money created in the local economy and the consequent recycling of that money within that local economy: 'when compared against cost per job estimates for a range of other government assistance programmes . . . it is a cost-effective way of creating jobs' (Fraser of Allander Institute 2001 and 2003).

Research carried out for the National Audit Office showed just how huge is the impact of both higher benefits and increased take-up among older people. The researchers concluded:

> In just one of our fieldwork sites (Cumbria), it appears that around £34 million per annum may be lost to the local economy as a result of non take-up of AA [Attendance Allowance] and MIG [Income Support] alone. This equates to approximately 800 jobs: a significant contribution to the rebuilding of a local economy which has been devastated by the impact of Foot and Mouth Disease.
>
> (Craig *et al.* 2002)

At an individual level, the same research highlighted the enormous impact of improved benefit take-up. Not only did people spend more on essentials, but also they enhanced their mobility, made use of goods and services (e.g. gardeners, hairdressers) which had previously been rationed due to lack of money and were able to purchase one-off items. The enhanced economic power led to a demonstrable enhanced level of physical independence, greater levels of participation, an improved sense of belonging, reaffirmed people's sense of identity and gave them a sense of dignity. One respondent stated:

'It has totally changed my life . . . it alters your whole outlook. If any problems arise you can cope with them'. (Craig *et al.* 2002, in National Audit Office 2002: 17–18).

One recent development by the Pension Service has been to promote the concept of joint teams between the Pension Service, local authorities and voluntary bodies with a unilateral government target of eventually having these in 100 per cent of local authorities. While superficially attractive, joint teams as envisaged by the Pension Service have a number of major operational, ethical and practical difficulties to overcome. Not least, the developments could have profound implications for welfare rights work – whether done by welfare rights specialists or by non-specialists and whether done by non-local authority bodies.

With the current fad for joining up public services, there is frequently an assumption that merging services produces better results. However, as one of the directors of Children's Services said:

> There is surprisingly little research literature about integrated multi-agency working, and nobody really knows whether it will ultimately prove more effective in supporting children's needs, and in terms of professional practice, than the more traditional professional silos model. To a large extent it is an article of faith that integrated team working will be better than non-integrated working.
>
> (Hawker 2005)

The same can be said of joint teams with the Pension Service.

The concept of a joint team is essentially that the DWP and local authorities and even voluntary organisations combine all their staff resources and all do the same work. Staff would share data, have the same conditions of service and provide help and advice (note: not advocacy) across the range of benefits and services that older people need. This allegedly enables them to provide a one-stop service to pensioners. Why this concept is limited to pensioners is unknown but the simplicity of the concept is compelling – particularly to those who are not familiar with advice work.

But the DWP's own internal organisational and benefit processes (for example, disability benefits administered by one office, Pension Credit by remote regional centres) mean that social security services themselves are highly fragmented and joint teams do nothing to weld these different internal organisations together. Even within joint teams, a huge amount of adviser time is spent trying to get one part of the DWP to communicate effectively with another part. Joint teams are an irrelevance to resolving the DWP's own barriers to take-up.

Even if it is the right thing to do, local authorities would do well to consider whether it is wise to partner so closely with an organisation which is the preferred point of contact for just 41 per cent of older people (Regional Centre for Neighbourhood Renewal 2004: 25).

The giving of advice on benefits is not a value-free or neutral activity and one's perspective is inevitably informed by a combination of professional values and the corporate values and priorities of one's employing body. Fundamental to welfare rights practice is the ability to act independently of the body one is advocating against and to be able to offer the best possible advice (in terms of options) to the client. Any service with the DWP is simply going to be unable to do this (and this is borne out by those local authorities which have joint teams).

The limitations of the role of benefit administrators as advice givers was highlighted by Fimister in 1986 and his analysis is still relevant:

> The view that, in the event of a disagreement over entitlement, the best person to advise the claimant is the other party to the dispute, is on the face of it so odd that it is surprising to find it so frequently held. I have described this elsewhere as 'roughly akin to asking a player in one of the teams at a football match to double as referee' (Fimister 1977: 8). David Bull has nevertheless 'encountered this position at a dangerously high level of social services management' (Bull 1982b: 11), in Bull's words (1982a: 6) . . . an 'especially facile argument'. But if such a view is so facile, why does it survive? The cause probably lies in a confusion between, on the one hand, the responsibility of benefit-administering agencies to publicise their wares and administer them efficiently; and on the other, the claimant's need for independent advice and support in the event of a problem or disagreement. This confusion is no doubt compounded by the fact that both welfare rights and benefit-administering agencies may engage in, and even collaborate over, benefit publicity exercises of one sort or another; while good liaison arrangements on individual cases may also convey a collaborative image. (This is indeed one of the drawbacks of the [DWP] 'liaison officer' system: it can lead the unwary to allow a friendly relationship to blunt a full insistence on the claimant's case.) For these reasons, there is a need to press home firmly the point that the [DWP] as a party to any potential disagreement, cannot provide independent advice and advocacy.
>
> (Fimister 1986: 18)

Such has been the scale of concern about joint teams that the National Association of Welfare Rights Advisers took the unprecedented step of issuing a Position Paper in 2005 which makes the point that: 'There is a key difference between administering benefits and advising people of their rights' and that:

> NAWRA recognises the importance of genuine partnership working . . . however we do not feel that Joint Teams amount to partnership working. We do not agree that they are the best model of service delivery and we feel that they threaten the existence of essential independent advice provision . . . Joint Teams are not in themselves likely to achieve huge increases in [benefits] take-up work. Local authorities should be aware that much successful take-up work involves a considerable amount of challenges at appeal so this independent function must be maintained.
>
> The most effective way to provide good welfare rights services is surely to be cooperative, to liase and to share information between agencies. But we must recognise that there needs to be a separation between those

providing welfare services and those deciding on access to benefits and financial support. To bring the operational functions too closely together means that roles can be compromised, the public can lose trust and the right to challenge decisions becomes severely diluted.

(National Association of Welfare Rights
Advisers 2005: 4–5)

For staff such as social workers, the development of a formal partnership with the DWP involving shared staffing also means that there be an increased likelihood that there will be an inherent reluctance to upset corporate partners by helping clients pursue the more robust legal remedies, effectively compromising their role as advocates – indeed some partnership agreements between local authorities and the DWP implicitly state this. There is also a danger that rather than empowering customers of local authorities, a joint team approach reinforces the paternalism of public services.

For welfare rights and advice services, the development of joint teams is a threat to their existence – it is all too easy for local authority decision makers to suggest or create a rationale for cuts in grants and services because 'the Pension Service now do this' and few such decision makers have a sufficient grasp of the difference between welfare rights work and benefits information giving and it is already resulting in cuts to welfare rights services.

However, even within its own terms the development of joint teams with local authorities means that the service focuses on local authority customers – about 4 per cent of all older people. While these can include some of the most marginalised members of society, it ignores the far wider cohort of older people living in poverty and who do not receive local authority services. As a result pension credit take-up could actually falter with such a strategy. In addition, joint teams do not provide a one-stop benefits service to older people because benefits are administered at several large centres, not by joint teams, and neither will joint teams provide help with appeals. Finally, one must question the value of such joint teams which are based on linking local authority charges for social care with benefits maximisation. In many cases, most of any additional disability benefits claimed with the help of a joint team are clawed back by the local authority, so the joint team is therefore operating more for the financial health of the local authority than for the customers. These arguments were set out in more detail in Bateman (2005).

Of even greater concern are signs that the unthinking rush to set up benefits information partnerships across the public sector is reaching lower down the age range, with the DWP's Jobcentre Plus service emerging as a partner in advice provision with local authorities.

While there is a positive and important role for appropriate partnership work on benefit take-up, such as data sharing and protocols for processing of claims, joint teams are not and cannot be a substitute for welfare rights practice.

Despite the concerns about how partnership work develops, the sanctioning by government of benefit take-up for children and older people can only be a good thing for welfare rights practice and can also be a way to secure additional funding for welfare rights services and activity.

NOT WELCOME HERE: MIGRATION AND SOCIAL SECURITY LAW

The history of social security mirrors the history of immigration controls by governments and the folk demon of the foreigner who comes to another country to scrounge handouts is as ancient and universal as the history of human migration and racism. There is no evidence that people who migrate are motivated by a desire to claim; indeed, it is often the case that migrants who are entitled, fail to claim because they are unaware of the existence and/or procedures for claiming. This is despite at least two pieces of recent research which show that migrants make fewer benefit claims than the indigenous population and that they also create a net gain in gross domestic product (for example, see Sriskandarajah *et al.* 2005).

Hostility to 'foreigners' has always manifested itself by either banning access to benefits or by resulting in sanctions for those who claim:

> The Secretary of State [for Health] may make an expulsion order respecting an alien who has not been in the United Kingdom for more than twelve months before proceedings are commenced, if he has within the previous three months been in receipt of poor law relief . . . The Merchant Shipping Act 1894 (s.185) enables the Secretary of State for India to take charge of and send home, or otherwise provide for, all lascars or natives of India who are found destitute in the United Kingdom.
>
> (Moss 1938: 65)

Over recent years we have found that benefits have been extensively restricted – cumulative bars preventing people seeking asylum from getting most benefits, banning access to those who are subject to immigration control, the introduction of the habitual residence test for claimants of means-tested benefits (and also access to public sector housing).

The habitual residence test was introduced in August 1994 following on from the infamous speeches by the then Secretary of State for Social Security, Peter Lilley, to the Conservative Party Conference in 1993, when he parodied French 'benefit tourists' asking '*Où est le Girocheque?*' There was little evidence that foreigners were coming to the UK for short periods and making benefit claims, though it was later alleged to me by a civil servant that an incident involving a young Italian man with a pet rat who visited a London social security office was the trigger for this ministerial moral panic. Inevitably, given its hasty and clumsy drafting and the lack of evidence of the need for the habitual residence test, the majority of people who have been refused benefit under the test have been British nationals returning to the UK.

A similar phenomenon of panic about foreigners milking the benefits system was experienced in 2004 with the hurried introduction of a 'right to reside' test for means-tested benefits. Introduced at short notice following a campaign in the tabloid press alleging that large numbers of people from the new eastern European member states (the 'A8') of the EU were preparing to present themselves at benefit offices in the UK

('Millions of migrants to flood in': front page headline in the *Daily Express* 19 February 2004), the rationale and design of the test was robustly criticised by the government's Social Security Advisory Committee in a detailed and scathing analysis:

> The adoption of a such a blanket approach at very short notice could in our view only be seen as appropriate and proportionate in the light of evidence that the UK's welfare benefits system is under substantial threat of exploitation by A8 nationals, or that the existing habitual residence test was demonstrably ineffective. We have been offered no evidence to support either assertion.
>
> (Social Security Advisory Committee 2004b: 25)

Almost predictably, the new test has affected many people who it was never designed to affect.

For those people who are subject to leave to remain (i.e. permission under the immigration rules) in the UK can find that just a simple enquiry about claiming means-tested benefits may result in their permission to remain in the UK being questioned or even rescinded.

Institutional racism also plays its part – continual difficulties about paying for interpreters in social security offices, the way that rules about identification and evidence of birth and marriage are operated, benefit rules which discriminate against Islamic mortgages, extended family living arrangements and traditional lending and borrowing arrangements which fall foul of means-tested benefit rules. These difficulties are exacerbated by what appears to be continual bad practice in many social security offices around basic matters such as a reluctance to use interpreters. One example I heard of concerned a Portuguese worker who was interviewed in Spanish by a DWP staff member who 'spoke some Spanish'; this is like a French speaker communicating in Danish with an English speaker on the basis that the latter two languages are related.

Not only among older first generation migrants into the UK, but even among second and third generation black and minority ethnic Britons, there is clear evidence of lower levels of benefit take-up alongside disproportionately higher levels of poverty and deprivation among many groups. This has even promoted an inquiry by the House of Commons Select Committee on Work and Pensions and research into the causes by the Department for Work and Pensions.

Financial and accommodation support schemes run by the Home Office to replace benefits for asylum seekers have not been without their problems and there is as much scope for advocacy about these rules in order to protect people as there is about benefits rules; indeed, the question about how far welfare rights advice should diversify into this area has been probed by at least one conference (Welfare Rights Advocacy: Issues and Barriers, CPAG, September 2004).

Questions of migration and race will continue to feature in the benefits system providing a clear need for welfare rights practitioners to act as advocates for socially unpopular groups and to challenge misapplication of already harsh and complicated rules as well as to challenge discriminatory procedures and attitudes. This is also an area where test cases flourish, for example the Collins decision of the European Court of

Justice which limited how the habitual residence test can be applied to unemployed EU jobseekers and challenges to force local authorities and the Home Office to support destitute asylum seekers.

ACTIVITY 2.2

What are the implications for public perceptions of the wider benefits system by the frequent focus on tightening benefits for people from abroad?

ALWAYS WITH US: THE PERSISTENCE OF SERIOUS LEVELS OF POVERTY AND INEQUALITY

Despite New Labour's positive measures to reduce poverty and unemployment, there remains a serious and widespread problem of poverty in the UK and this is at a time when wealth inequality has continued to widen.

The growth in inequality in New Labour's earlier years means that people in the poorest groups are increasingly left behind and excluded and the experience of poverty becomes even more difficult for them.

Part of the government's response to poverty and inequality has been to establish the Social Exclusion Unit within central government to analyse and advise on policy. However, rather than focusing on poverty as a whole and examining the ways it affects people, the unit has chosen to focus on a number of effects of poverty (such as the educational attainment of children in care and the exclusionary effects of mental illness):

> Social exclusion is about more than income poverty. Social exclusion happens when people or places suffer from a series of problems such as unemployment, discrimination, poor skills, low incomes, poor housing, high crime, ill health and family breakdown. When such problems combine they can create a vicious cycle. Social exclusion can happen as a result of problems that face one person in their life. But it can also start from birth. Being born into poverty or to parents with low skills still has a major influence on future life chances.
>
> (Social Exclusion Unit 2004a)

Because of tensions between government departments (e.g. the desire of policy makers in the DWP to reduce the number receiving sickness-related benefits, clashing with the desire of those in the Department of Health to address ill health) some of the Social Exclusion Unit's reports have completely avoided addressing deficiencies in the social security system. For example:

The benefits system should provide financial support and underpin security
when people with mental health problems are unwell and unable to work.
But evidence from advice bureaux shows that too often it does just the
reverse . . . by sidestepping these issues it [Social Exclusion Unit report
Mental Health and Social Exclusion 2004] fails to create the building blocks
of positive experience when people are unwell which might help their
recovery.

(Cullen 2004)

Benefit recommendations in another unit report, *Bridging the Gap: New Opportunities
for 16–18 Year Olds Not in Education, Employment or Training*, gathered dust on
DWP policy section shelves for three years after its publication in 1999 until a coalition
of interest groups working tactically with the unit succeeded in getting ministerial
attention to focus on the need for reform of the system of financial support for young
people, which is starting to produce some positive modifications.

An unfortunate side-effect is that the use of the term 'social exclusion' has obscured
the debate about poverty and acted as a distraction. This term was originally popularised
as a political compromise within the European Community in the 1980s because
of objections from the British, French and German governments to the use of the word
'poverty' in official publications and funding criteria. 'Social Exclusion's modern usage
is more political than sociological in origin' (Lister 2004: 75) and there is little research
or objective evidence to underpin the concept.

The accepted position about the definition of poverty had always been Townsend's
definition, based on extensive data and empirical research, that income poverty leads
to exclusion from 'ordinary living patterns, customs and activities' (Townsend 1979:
31). However, repeated (and frequently ill-informed) use of the phrase 'social exclusion'
in the public sector has meant that the income and inequality dimension and origins
are often ignored and the fundamental causes of social exclusion are not adequately
acknowledged. If they were, a very different approach would result with less emphasis
on personal pathology. It also means that groups which are deemed to experience
social exclusion include people who are wealthy, for example, the British Royal Family
are socially excluded from mainstream society. Equally, people experiencing poverty
can live in very inclusive communities, thus posing 'a challenge to the concept of "social
exclusion"' (Page 2000: 46, cited in Lister 2004: 85).

As discussed in Chapter 1, the late 1970s and 1980s saw a huge growth in inequality
and poverty. The Gini Coefficient, which is an accepted standard method of measuring
income and wealth inequality, leapt from 25 per cent to 34 per cent, demonstrating an
increase in inequality of 40 per cent. Since 1997, despite improvements in incomes for
the poorest (in large part due to economic growth: Brewer *et al.* 2004) inequality has
continued to rise and then only fall slightly (2003–04 Gini Coefficient was 33.9 per cent).
This is perhaps inevitable given the fundamental economic and social changes which the
policies of the previous 20 years brought about and the resulting exponential impact of
economic growth on income growth among the rich:

over the 1980s, there was a considerable increase in inequality as measured
by the Gini Coefficient. It stabilised in the early 1990s, and then fell slightly

over the last Conservative government. Since Labour came to power, the Gini Coefficient has increased once more. Indeed, despite the slight (statistically insignificant) fall in 2001–02, income inequality over the past two years has been higher than in any other period covered by our data.

(Shephard 2003: 4)

Among the major industrialised countries, the UK now ranks second to the USA in inequality.

The Labour Party is now 'intensely relaxed about people getting filthy rich', argued Peter Mandelson in a speech to Silicon Valley executives, while Tony Blair famously refused to say that he cared about the gap between rich and poor when interviewed before the 2001 general election.

(Jackson and Segal 2004: 7)

As discussed earlier, the scale of poverty has diminished slightly since 1997:

- In 2001/02, 12.5 million people in Great Britain (22 percent of the population) were living in households with below 60 percent of median income after housing costs.
- At the end of 1999, 14.5 million people in Great Britain (26 percent) were living in poverty according to the PSA survey, (defined as lacking two or more socially perceived necessities), a comparison with earlier Breadline Britain surveys shows that in 1983, 14 percent of households lacked three or more socially perceived necessities rising by 1990 to 21 percent and by 1999 to over 24 percent.

(Flaherty et al. 2004: 31)

- The most commonly used threshold of low income is 60 per cent of median income. In 2002/03, before deducting housing costs, this equated to £194 per week for a couple with no children, £118 for a single person, £283 for a couple with two children and £207 for a lone parent with two children.
- In 2002/03, 12.4 million people were living on incomes below this income threshold. This represents a drop of 1.5 million since 1996/97.
- The numbers of people on relative low incomes remained broadly unchanged during the 1990s after having doubled in the 1980s.
- In 2002/03, there were 8 million people on incomes below the fixed threshold of 60 per cent of 1996/97 median income. This represents a drop of 6 million since 1996/97.

(www.poverty.org.uk)

While the progress on reducing poverty may well be maintained through government attention, albeit at different rates among different groups, it could be reversed if inequality does not reduce further and it still has a long way to go before it is reduced even to levels of the mid-1970s – even then there was more than enough welfare rights work to be done in an era when the scale of means testing was less and with less scope for disputes as a result.

An accompanying issue is the growth and extent of debt among people on low incomes. Within inadequate benefit levels and a state-run loans system for one-off payments (the Social Fund – even though loans are interest free, repayments are at a higher rate than commercial loans) many benefit claimants turn to lenders for help. Debt has a highly damaging effect on health and well-being (e.g. 'The impact of unmanageable debt on an individual's life can be overwhelming': Edwards 2003: 4). It also acts as a barrier to entering work (because creditors demand increased repayments) and is also associated with relationship breakdown and child neglect and abuse. The UK has one of the least regulated credit industries in the western world and vigorous informal and formal credit sectors which frequently target people on low incomes (witness the mass of credit advertisements in tabloid newspapers) and overall personal debt levels have been rising.

The incidence of debt and low income is well established. For example:

- A third of households with incomes less than £900 a year have debts
- 33% of local authority and housing association tenants have rent arrears compared to 8% of home owners with mortgage debt
- Nearly half of all lone parents had been in arrears with housing costs in the past year
- Unemployed households were more than twice as likely (43%) to have experienced arrears than those with one or more members in full-time employment.

(Flaherty *et al.* 2004: 115–18)

The survey also found that certain debts were linked to poverty. Women, tenants of social landlords and the unwaged were most likely to have debts associated with poverty, such as catalogue debts and loans to home-collected credit providers. Interest rates associated with these types of borrowing were significantly greater than for so-called mainstream sources of credit.

(Edwards 2003)

Welfare rights practice can help manage debt problems and sometimes completely eliminate them (for example, many housing debts are entirely caused by benefit problems and errors). The growth of debt, sadly, looks as if it will fuel a need for welfare rights work for many years to come as well as being a huge source of need for specialist advice in itself and wider awareness among people working in the voluntary and public sectors, who are often the first to be contacted by people in debt. And there is strong evidence that debt and benefit problems are not discrete, tidy packages but are usually a bundle of interrelated benefit, debt and rented housing issues (Legal Services Commission 2004: 40). There is a case for welfare rights practitioners also building on their expertise in debt advice, or at least having sufficient knowledge and strong links in order to make informed referrals. Debt advisers may also need to consider their level of expertise in income maximisation as part of the debt advice process – the debate needs to occur.

To exacerbate the scale and experience of poverty, benefit take-up levels remain a problem and, indeed, in some cases, the level of take-up has worsened since 1997 as the qualifying income levels of means-tested benefits have risen, bringing more people into entitlement – an unintended consequence of a benign social policy.

BOX 2.1:   THE TAKE-UP CHALLENGE

Benefit	Take-up rate (percentage of those entitled and receiving)	No. of entitled non-recipients
Income support (pensioners)	63–74%	870,000
Income support (non-pensioners)	85–95%	350,000
Pension credit	66%	1 million
Housing benefit	84–90%	680,000
Council tax benefit	65–71%	2.34 million
Attendance allowance	40–60%	N/A
Disability living allowance	30–50% (care component)	N/A
	50–70% (mobility component)	

Sources: DWP 2005; National Audit Office 2002

Other estimates show that among some groups (e.g. pensioners entitled to council tax benefit only), take-up runs at just 44 per cent (Hancock *et al.* 2004: 298) and non-claiming local authority and housing association tenants who are pensioners are underclaiming and thus 'forgoing income supplements averaging 41 per cent of their income' (Hancock *et al.* 2004: 298).

Even among people with a terminal illness, where rules of entitlement to disability living allowance and attendance allowance have been massively simplified and which are specially administered on a very fast track service, research for the cancer support charity, the Macmillan Foundation, has indicated that take-up is not at the levels one would hope it was, with 54 per cent of all people with a terminal cancer diagnosis not receiving the benefits they were entitled to (Tunnage *et al.* 2004).

By contrast, the less complex non-means-tested benefits, such as retirement pension and child benefit, effectively have take-up rates of 100 per cent.

The persistence of poor benefit take-up rates and persistence of poverty provides a strong business case and socio-economic driver for welfare rights practice.

Not only do most of those who feature in the poverty statistics rely on means-tested benefits as their main source of income, but also improving take-up of benefits among poorer people is a direct way of addressing poverty and the resulting social exclusion and anyone who works with people who experience poverty is likely to find that they have to deal with that poverty in order to solve other problems and welfare rights practice is a practical and empowering response.

Alongside tackling underclaiming and ironing out errors, there is the important work done by welfare rights practitioners to challenge benefits sanctions. Sadly, few people seek help when they are sanctioned and DWP figures show that a dispro-portionate number of young people and people from black and minority ethnic backgrounds have their benefits cut or reduced by sanctions. New Labour is committed to the big stick approach inherent in sanctions; indeed it has increased the number of 'offences' for which people can be sanctioned. However, sanctioning has other effects, such as deterring people from engaging with the system and thus not getting support they qualify for, and increasing crime:

> In April 2004 a University College of London study demonstrated a link between claimants disappearing from the register due to sanctions and 2–3 per cent increase in crime. Apply sanctions to those with chaotic lifestyles as a result, for example, of homelessness or drug and alcohol problems, and they are driven off both benefits and [training] schemes and back onto the streets and crime.
>
> (Holmes 2005: 11)

Welfare rights advocacy and lobbying can therefore contribute to wider economic and social well-being.

GROWING BY THE DAY: INCREASING NUMBERS OF OLDER PEOPLE

Older people are major users of the social security system and as discussed, a growing number of them are entitled to means-tested benefits to top up their pensions and require help to access their full entitlement. In addition, the complex relationship between social

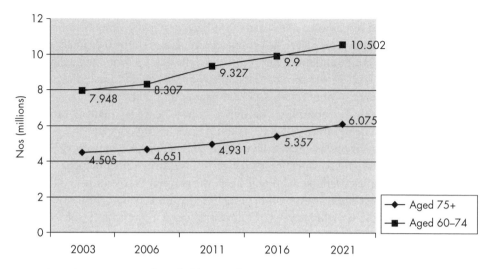

Figure 2.2 The growing number of older people
Source: Shaw 2004: 13

security and social care services means that welfare rights help will be increasingly required unless there is a profound change in all the main political parties social policies – such as the introduction of a non-means-tested Citizens Income Scheme for older people.

The number of older people is growing and the number of elderly older people (who are poorer) is growing even more. The data in Figure 2.2 are self-explanatory.

In addition, we can expect to see life expectancy rise by over three years by 2021 to 79.9 years for men and 83.9 for women and a fall in the support ratio of working age people to over sixties from 3.34 in 2003 to 3.15 in 2021 and 2.87 in 2026 (Shaw 2004: 13). Despite this demographers suggest that there is 'considerable uncertainty regarding the future size of the population' (Shaw 2004: 14). Potentially migration and changes in working patterns could alter the population structure thus making good falling support ratios (which in turn has implications for social security policy as discussed earlier).

SOME DIE SOONER: HEALTH INEQUALITIES

There are proven links between poverty and ill health, with men in Social Class V dying seven years earlier then those in Social Class I (Flaherty *et al.* 2004: 124; Acheson 1998). The evidence about links between poverty and ill health is longstanding and irrefutable:

> Note: most of the statistics below relate to the year 2002, the latest year for which official data currently exists.

- Scotland has by far the highest proportion of premature deaths for both men and women.
- Adults in the poorest fifth of the income distribution are twice as likely to be at risk of developing a mental illness as those on average incomes.
- Almost half of adults aged 45–64 in the poorest fifth of the population have a limiting longstanding illness or disability, twice the rate for those on average incomes.
- Children from manual social backgrounds are 1½ times more likely to die as infants than children from non-manual social backgrounds.
- Babies from manual social backgrounds are 1⅓ times more likely to be of low birthweight than those from non-manual social backgrounds.
- Teenage motherhood is six times as common amongst those from manual social backgrounds as for those from professional backgrounds.
- 5-year-olds in Scotland, Wales and North West have, on average, twice as many missing, decayed or filled teeth as 5-year-olds in the West Midlands and South East.

(www.poverty.org.uk)

There are numerous reasons why poverty leads to worse health, for example worse diet, greater stress levels, worse housing, more dangerous work, lower educational attainment, higher levels of smoking. Lack of enough money will inevitable mean that these risk enhancing factors are exacerbated.

Epidemiologist Richard Wilson (1993) has taken the analysis further and demonstrated that societies which have greater levels of inequality tend to have higher levels of social competitiveness and lower levels of communality. The long-term stress related and other effects of this are evidenced as key causes of ill health. Consequently a poor child born in inner city USA has a shorter life expectancy than a poor child born in rural Bangladesh.

People on low incomes are also more likely to require more expensive forms of health care, partly because they have less access to preventative health care and thus are more likely to require hospitalisation. There is a strong economic and health service efficiency case for reducing the impact of poverty on ill health (and by reducing ill health through poverty reduction) and it also recognises that in recent years better medical understanding and diagnosis has brought about new customers for welfare rights services – for example, children with attention hyperactivity disorder, people with autistic spectrum disorders and the growth of stress-related illnesses.

The co-location of welfare rights advice in health settings (as well as recommendations for increases in means-tested benefits) was a specific recommendation in the government sponsored Acheson (1998) report and since then there has been a continual process of developing these services. In particular, devolved powers in Wales led to the Welsh Assembly in 2003 agreeing to fund independent welfare rights services in all Welsh primary care services.

Additional income reduces health problems – for example, American research in Indiana showed that after equivalising for other factors, mothers who received higher levels of means-tested benefits had babies with higher birthweights compared to mothers who received lower levels. This is a significant finding because low birthweight is a key determinant of future health problems and disability throughout life (Kehrer and Wolin 1979), while research in San Francisco showed that introducing a higher level for minimum wages reduces sickness levels and early deaths among people of working age (Bhatia and Katz 2001).

Welfare rights work allied to health care is one practical response to the links between poverty and ill health. Not only does it improve people's income levels so that their risk factors are improved, but also its rights nature and one-to-one basis may have a 'Hawthorn Effect' (the unexpected promotion of positive behaviour as result of personal attention by another). In addition, primary health care practitioners frequently see the results of poverty and ill health and are increasingly (by stealth) being used as gatekeepers to the benefits system by the DWP – with obvious implications for their values and attitudes and which may challenge their traditional role as advocates for their patients.

With the government emphasising the need to address health inequalities (and indeed, this being essential to secure any step change in overall health improvement statistics), increasing numbers of welfare rights services linked to health care have been developed since 1997; indeed, it has probably been the main growth area in recent years. No cross-agency surveys have been done, but one might estimate that there are now many hundreds of welfare rights advisers working in health care settings. They operate alongside professionals such as health-based social workers, many of whom have traditionally acted as a first point of call on benefit problems for patients.

There is considerable research evidence to show the health improving effects of welfare rights advice, with at least 21 research reports in the UK alone and numerous other reports about health-based welfare advice (many of which are summarised in Greasley and Small 2002). A typical finding is that primary health care advice targeted at people who have chronic health problems produces a 'statistically significant health gain . . . an important association between those patients who had an increase in income' (Vaux 2000; Abbott and Hobby 1999, 2000). The same research demonstrated a reduction in demand for help from general practitioners (GPs) from patients whose income had been increased because of welfare rights advice and 69 per cent of this group reported improvements in their health and well-being. The funding of welfare rights advisers in primary health care across all of Wales by the Welsh Assembly showed that in 2002–03 up to 91.3 per cent of clients who had received advice felt better (none felt worse!) and 62.5 per cent of participating GPs felt that patients' general health had been improved by this service (Borland 2004: 13 and 19).

By late 2004, it was estimated (Citizens Advice 2004b) that among just Citizens Advice Bureaux in England and Wales, advice services were located in 751 general practice clinics and health centres, 62 general hospitals and 165 mental health clinics (mostly part time). The number of welfare rights advice sessions run by local authorities in health care settings is unknown (but probably at least as large as the Citizens Advice Bureaux) and if one includes the health-based social workers who give welfare rights advice, the number is huge. Despite the emphasis on public health improvements designed to address inequalities, these services have developed 'on a piecemeal, ad hoc basis and Primary Care Trusts offer no such services at all' (Citizens Advice 2004b).

The location of welfare rights specialists within health care opens up exciting . opportunities to reach out to a cohort of people who do not make use of other services (Abbott and Hobby 2003), to target benefits advice and advocacy at people with pressing health needs and to also develop welfare rights knowledge and skills among medical and nursing practitioners. Some welfare rights advisers have taken matters further by trawling patient databases in primary health care in order to identify groups of underclaimers (for example, those with restricted mobility or who are aged over 80 or people with particular disabilities which attract particular benefits, such as people who have had work related accidents and diseases) and to target appropriate infor- mation at them. Work has also been done by health-based welfare rights advisers to improve training and knowledge of health professionals and to work with doctors to help them better manage the burden of providing evidence for benefit claims by ensuring that evidence which is provided is concise, relevant and well presented.

It seems that the taking of well-targeted referrals in primary health care settings is a source of great success – Lancashire County Council's Welfare Rights Service helped half of all patients referred to its specialist advisers to claim extra benefits (Vaux 2000) and in Wakefield 57 per cent of those seen made successful benefit claims (Lishman-Peat and Brown 2002), while across all of Wales, £3.44 million in additional was claimed in 2002–03 by health-based welfare rights advisers (Borland 2004: 10).

However, even though the National Health Service now places greater emphasis on the socio-economic factors of ill health and even though local authorities have developed a locus on health care, secure and sustainable funding remains a problem for many health-based welfare rights advisers. Health service resource allocators can sometimes see welfare rights work as not 'real health care' and local authorities can see it as 'a health problem'. And both will readily provide a long list of urgent funding needs within their core services.

While some external funding may be possible (for example via charities or the Legal Services Commission), this is also not without its drawbacks (see Chapter 3 for a fuller discussion of funding options).

Such issues highlight that health-based welfare rights practice is still in the growth phase.

ACTIVITY 2.3

From your own practice, identify opportunities for linking welfare rights practice with health services.

A SAFE HOME? WELFARE RIGHTS AND HOUSING

Any adviser who has dealt with rent arrears problems soon realises that the solution frequently lies in resolving a benefits problem, for example a delay or error in housing benefit, or with another benefit or a failure to claim benefits which the debtor is entitled to. So it makes sound sense for social landlords to invest in welfare rights expertise as a cheaper and less painful remedy than automatically reaching for the harsh and punitive remedies of court action.

While social work professionals long ago realised the value of welfare rights advice as a way of helping them do their work, the message has taken far longer to be acknowledged by housing providers – with a few notable exceptions.

One early pioneer in linking welfare rights advice to prevention of rent arrears and homelessness was Liverpool City Council, with a team dedicated to doing such work. Within two years the team produced benefit gains of £718,027 (mostly translated into reduced rent arrears) over and above the cost of setting up and running the service (Craven 2000).

A major development was the decision by the Audit Commission Housing Inspectorate (2001) to include examining the provision of advice on debt and welfare rights as part of its routine inspections of social landlords. Since then social landlords have been marked up or down (and publicly) depending on the extent and availability of welfare rights advice to tenants who are having difficulty paying their rent. However, reading the reports, it is unclear how thorough and how consistent the inspections are on this point (apparently being carried out by non-welfare rights experts). But this measure has undoubtedly led not only to the direct employment of welfare rights advisers or the provision of such help under contract to mainstream advice agencies but also to improved levels of benefits training and awareness among housing staff generally.

Unfortunately there are no figures to show the number of such specialist posts within social landlords and welfare rights advisers employed by such bodies also report that there is often a tension between their role as advocates and income maximisers and the staff who are responsible for managing rent arrears who take amore punitive, traditional approach. They can also feel like income raisers for the organisation rather than advisers with a duty towards a client. A probable solution lies in developing specialist posts as second tier advisers – the advantages of this are discussed later in this chapter.

WELFARE RIGHTS PRACTICE BY SOCIAL WORKERS

The involvement by practitioners such as social workers in welfare rights work is long and distinguished and as discussed in Chapter 1, social workers were instrumental in establishing the modern welfare rights movement in the 1970s.

Welfare rights practice fits neatly with the central task of social work, which is to empower and protect vulnerable and/or marginalised individuals and in practical terms. And because over 90 per cent of social work service users receive means-tested benefits, dealing with and managing the consequences of their money problems are everyday realities for social workers. Welfare rights work is therefore an unavoidable activity which has featured as a part of social work practice to some extent or another since the earliest days of the social work profession. It is no coincidence that many local authority welfare rights services are located within social services departments.

In this section, while referring to social workers, I am also including the wider group of social care professionals and employees, many of whom have a hands-on and practical role which can bring them closer to the people who use care services.

Social workers are often asked for help with financial problems not only because they have residual income maintenance powers but also because they are perceived as being able to resolve benefit problems and to bring the authority of their employing organisation into the process (which places them at an advantage over voluntary bodies). In 1979, Goldberg and Warburton's study of incoming problems to social work teams in Southampton found that financial problems made up 17 per cent of all referrals, the second highest category of problems which were presented.

Poverty lies at the heart of many of the issues which social workers deal with – when presented as a discrete financial problem, as part of a package of issues or when it is worsening another problem or even causing it. This is not to say that poverty inevitably leads to child neglect and abuse or a need for community services nor that people mistreat their children just because they are poor – the vast majority of people living on low incomes are as caring parents as anyone else. It is simply summarising the evidence that poverty makes it a lot more difficult to navigate significant life vents and the ups and downs of everyday experiences.

However, while almost all people in social work recognise the significance of poverty and inequality, it does not readily overtly influence professional practice. One observational study concluded: 'Social workers appear aware of poverty in theory and acknowledge it is an indisputable part of social services users' lives. In practice the fieldwork has suggested they appear to find it difficult to translate attitudes into actions' (Dowling 1999: 162). A similar view based on observation was put by Green: 'at the individual level, social workers appear to be suffering from collective amnesia as to why most of us came into the social work profession in the first place' (Green 2000). Another similar view was expressed by Becker:

> Many social workers have distanced themselves traditionally from the material and cash problems of their clients, which if they are acknowledged at all, are seen as the proper responsibilities of other agencies, particularly the social security bureaucracies, or other specialist such as welfare rights advisers. While many social work users are claimants of social security, and many are also poor, this does not translate itself into prescriptions for social services policy or social work practice . . . social services and social workers have largely managed poor families with children by defining them as dysfunctional families requiring individual or family treatment, rather than

confronting and engaging with poverty as a structural and political issue. The social work 'mission' has centred on helping individuals to function more effectively in their social environment.

(Becker 1997: 93 and 113)

The issues which are related to poverty include the increased incidence of disability and ill health (both mental and physical), the greater incidence of relationship stress and breakdown (Yeandle *et al.* 2003), the greater chance of being a victim of crime (Pullinger and Summerfield 1999) and the exclusion from hobbies and social activities (Gordon *et al.* 2000). Poverty leads to 'loss of self esteem, anger, depression, anxiety and boredom . . . many spoke of its damaging effects on personal relationships and the way it stigmatised people . . . restricting people's opportunities and choices and making budgeting a never ending tyranny' (Beresford *et al.* 1999, cited in Davies 2002: 133). As already mentioned, there is even evidence from the USA that increased levels of means-tested benefits improve babies' birthweights – a key predictor of future health and life chances.

Evidence has long existed about the strong correlation between debts, unemployment and placement of a child on the Child Protection Register (National Children's Homes 1986; Becker and MacPherson 1986; Irvine 1986; Baldwin and Spencer 1993) and the disproportionate incidence of children who enter the care system coming from the poorest families (for example, see Freeman and Lockhart 1994; Department of Health 1995). A more detailed examination can be found in Becker (1997).

The marginalisation of poverty as an issue which social work can play a part in addressing has been further accelerated by the emphasis in government guidance about charges for care services. This guidance – for example, the Department of Health's *Fairer Charging Policies for Home Care . . . Practice Guidance* (Department of Health 2002) – rightly emphasises the need to maximise the incomes of those service users who are liable to pay charges for their care services:

Councils should ensure that appropriate benefits advice is provided to all users of non-residential social services and carers services at the time of a charge assessment . . . any charge assessment should be focused on the user's overall finances and personal needs. It will normally need to be carried out by personal interview in the user's own home by appropriately skilled staff. The service should include advice about entitlement, help with completion of benefit claims and follow-up action, if the user wishes.

(Department of Health 2002: 21)

However, by placing income maximisation within the context of revenue generation for the local authority, there has been a noticeable shift by many social services departments to concentrate their welfare rights resources at this, operationally, minor end of their functions at the expense of other areas. This inevitably leads to a decline in welfare rights awareness across the organisation and particularly disadvantages the large number of service users who do not receive chargeable care services (for example, children and families, which is somewhat irrational given the government's pledge to end child poverty).

Welfare rights practice can add value to social work practice in many ways:

- It is a practical response to service users who have money problems.
- It addresses some of the underlying problems which create a need for social work.
- The additional income helps people to live more independent lives.
- Resolving financial issues can often be required before clients are able to successfully engage with other forms of interventions.
- It can reduce expenditure under the residual income maintenance functions of social work organisations such as duties to provide exceptional financial support to keep children out of the care system or financial support for young people who have left the care system.
- It builds trust, empathy and a dialogue with service users by the worker being seen to deal with a pressure point in their lives and responding to what they see as a high priority need. It helps people to feel valued.
- The rights-based perspective empowers service users which can lead to improvements to other aspects of their coping ability and enables worker and client to operate on a less unequal basis, thus empowering the client.
- The task-based approach inherent in welfare rights practice can complement task-based social work techniques.
- Extra money from disability benefits is used by recipients on services which are analogous to community care services – it appears that 25 per cent of disability living allowance care component is spent in this way (Noble *et al.* 1997).
- For those social care services which are chargeable, additional benefits can directly lead to extra income for the local authority. Additional disability benefits also positively affect the government's grant formula (the Formula Spending share) for a local authority with a higher level of take-up, welfare rights advice can avoid pitfalls when making payments to service users for consultation activities, and helping local authorities to avoid using their own funds to support people who should be accessing benefits, for example, care-leavers, destitute families and people affected by the habitual residence test.
- There are requirements on social services to provide information and help about welfare rights is clarified in several government guidance documents – such as guidance on aftercare for people who are compulsorily treated under mental health legislation and the National Service Framework for Children and Young People.
- It improves the money supply within low income communities, thus aiding wider economic regeneration.
- If properly supported and resourced, many social workers find this an enjoyable area of work which contrasts to their other roles as social controllers and resource gatekeepers.
- Social work professionals work with some of the most marginalised people, who may not be able to sustain contact or even access mainstream welfare rights advice services.

Sadly almost no research has been carried out on the positive effects of integrating welfare rights work and social work practice; it would be a useful area to develop and to gather better evidence.

Despite the strong case for welfare rights practice by social work professionals, there has always been a degree of ambivalence about its place and this ambivalence often increases, the higher up the long hierarchy that one ascends. Inevitably, one's own values and attitudes towards money, poverty and the politics of welfare are subconscious influences which are frequently overlooked (which highlights the importance of a non-judgemental approach). This personal influence has been discussed by Ryan (1996) in relation to social work with people in debt and was developed into a self-assessment exercise by Fook (1993). Fook's self-assessment exercise includes getting social workers to ask themselves (either in a group or individually), asking what money means to them, where these attitudes come from, how they feel about being in debt and how these attitudes influence their perceptions of and work with people living in poverty. Such an exercise could, of course, be applied to many other professionals.

The argument against welfare rights practice by social workers seems to usually involve the following points:

- There is not enough time to do it.
- It is a specialist area and beyond the individual social worker's knowledge base (even if they knew it originally).
- It is adversarial.
- It is the responsibility of another agency.

When examined, these views are frequently based on a poor understanding of what welfare rights work involves. They are the types of view frequently put forward by people who have invariably undertaken welfare rights work with insufficient support, advice and resources, which all makes for an unsatisfactory experience. It is indisputable that there are huge pressures on social workers' time for doing welfare rights and many other things, but it is vital that resource constraints are not allowed to turn (or be used as an excuse to turn) social work into a minimalist, statutory function-based activity if it is to retain any support and credibility among service users.

Yes, it can be a specialist area, just as mental health social work is, but social workers have to know about mental health issues, without becoming experts, even if they do not work in the mental health field.

The key to finding the time to do welfare rights work and also to manage the more detailed aspects is having sufficient support and back-up – for example by having an in-house, second tier welfare rights service to provide advice training and to take on complex cases and also by having ready access to the service and being provided with basic resources (such as reference books) in order to do the job.

In terms of its adversarialism, yes advocacy may be adversarial, but advocacy per se is a fundamental part of the social work role. For example, the Code of Practice for Social Care Workers includes a requirement that social care workers 'must protect the rights and promote the interests of service users and carers' and that they should promote 'the independence of service users and assist them to understand and exercise their rights', including helping 'service users and carers to make complaints' and finally to 'respect the rights of service users' (General Social Care Council 2004). Or, in more therapeutic terms: 'Strategies of change in social work might sometimes need to be directed, not at the client, but at dysfunctional elements in the client's environment' (Davies 1994).

It is also helpful to clarify that welfare rights work is a continuum. It is not necessary for everyone to operate at the most complex end of this continuum and much valuable work can be done by less skilled advisers. Advice work generally has been classified as having three levels of complexity (see page 97). It is unrealistic to expect social workers or other non-specialists to operate at the more complex levels, but they can at the less complex levels.

The ability to enforce rights is a fundamental part of our democracy and of holding the state to account and having senior managers in social care agencies confirm the role of staff as advocates with those agencies which find this uncomfortable is a vital step in managing and reducing the resulting tensions. Simply pretending that advocacy will go away does not work. Where this becomes much more difficult to manage is when social care organisations enter into formal partnerships with income maintenance organisations – see the earlier discussion about the implications of joint teams with the Pension Service.

The view that welfare rights work is the responsibility of another agency does not fit with the increasing emphasis on seamless services and while specialist level welfare rights work (for example tribunal representation) is a specialist function; even if such work is to be done by another body, social work staff still need a critical mass of benefits knowledge in order to know when and what to refer. Suffice it to say, even a highly customer-orientated Department for Work and Pensions would not be able to operate as a welfare rights service. As mentioned earlier, some of the people whom social workers support are not able to work with other agencies and may fall foul of their rules about 'client cooperation'. In practical terms, if social workers did not do any welfare rights work, it would leave a huge gap.

Welfare rights services within social care agencies have often succeeded in supporting social work practitioners to undertake welfare rights work and by developing realistic levels of competence in welfare rights work. An appropriate level of competence in welfare rights work might include the following:

- being able to identify benefit and tax credit entitlement in common situations
- helping people through the claims process, providing supporting evidence and resolving common problems which can arise
- acting as an advocate to resolve common problems and successfully challenging straightforward benefit refusals
- protecting clients from inappropriate questioning or investigation by benefit officials
- attempting to modify negative or stereotyped attitudes among benefit officials who they deal with
- supporting a vulnerable service user though an appeal with representation being done by a welfare rights specialist.

Since the 1990s, social work in the UK has come under increasing public scrutiny (amplified by scapegoating press coverage) as a result of a number of high profile service failures. This has led to an increased emphasis on systems, external inspection and performance improvement measures imposed by central government. Since 1993, there has also been a strong emphasis on business principles and processes with social workers care managing and purchasing packages of care to a defined specification and operating nationally defined eligibility criteria to determine access to services.

While a more structured and strategic approach was needed for the delivery of social care, and while social work skills remain very relevant, particularly when assessing people's needs for services, there is a perception that many of the more creative skills and activities (including welfare rights practice) have been marginalised by these processes, and welfare rights work, if done at all frequently, can been seen simply as a revenue-raising activity. Despite this, there remains a strong interest in welfare rights practice among many social workers; large amounts of their time are spent undertaking such work and they are also a key source of referrals to specialist welfare rights services.

The development of joint teams between the DWP and local authorities will not and is not designed to engage social workers in welfare rights work and they are likely to further reduce their engagement in areas where joint teams are set up.

A number of local authorities (for example, Manchester, Suffolk and Newham) have achieved praise from external inspectorates for the way in which they have taken steps to integrate welfare rights work in social services settings and for linking it to strategic corporate priorities, such as helping people move into jobs, supporting services for care leavers or helping people discharged from hospital.

Continuing to reinvigorate social workers' interest and engagement in welfare rights work is part of the process of helping social work practitioners keep in touch with their professional roots while also ensuring welfare rights practice fits with and adds value to the changed social work environment – particularly as social care services become fragmented into separate child- and adult-based organisations.

What does not work in social work practice (or any other area outside welfare rights practice) is the concept of nominating one team member to be an expert – they hold the books, attend training course and then feedback to others. Experience shows that this can result in the 'expert' being overloaded (thus embedding the marginalisation of welfare rights practice) and the technical nature of welfare tights tends to overwhelm the feedback process. Because it is so limited as a learning method, one would not apply this to any mainstream area of work, so why to welfare rights practice?

Practical ways to achieve this are discussed further in this chapter and in Chapter 3.

ACTIVITY 2.4

What are the implications for social work practice if all welfare rights awareness and practice is removed?

WE'RE ALL MANAGERS NOW

The development of managerial expertise within the public sector since the 1990s has affected welfare rights practice as much as any other area of public service. One advantage is that compared to most other public services, it is easy to measure outcomes and outputs from welfare rights work and to make meaningful comparisons between different models of delivery because one can often measure the benefit gained from welfare rights advice and advocacy. There is also substantial research evidence about the positive effects of increased benefits take-up; indeed, it is a far more researched area than many other areas of public service.

The case for welfare rights practice, either as part of other work by non-specialists or as part of a case for funding dedicated specialists, is frequently made using benefit gain figures and many areas have been able to preserve welfare rights provision when decision makers have been faced with robust evidence about the outcomes.

Despite this there are no standardised measures of benefit gains and different agencies use different methods, some of which are of questionable accuracy while some use inquiry-based outputs which can easily be mistaken for a headcount-based approach. In part this reflects the inherent dilemma of any performance management system – measure something to find an answer and you end up with more questions. Management is an art and not a science which means that the concepts and approaches are imperfect, but they are less imperfect than approaches to running organisations which are based on informal or traditional 'ways of doing things'.

The implication of the more professionalised approach to managing services is that welfare rights work has to be justified in hard objective terms alongside other activities competing for time or resources, consequently welfare rights specialists have had to rethink their approach to service delivery:

> Welfare rights services have had to move from being open-door informal advice services for claimants to being highly organised services which seek to influence a range of key stakeholders. However, the original ethos and objectives of welfare rights work remain unchanged . . . the obligation to deliver excellence is going to be increasingly important . . . we have tended to under-manage welfare rights advice services, partly out of a sentimental attachment to confused and naïve anti-establishments political philosophies.
>
> (Patterson 2001)

Even if many front line workers resent it, the increased managerial atmosphere of public services will not go away. The trick is to use the best aspects of it to preserve and enhance the unique usefulness of welfare rights practice.

Allied to the changed management culture of the late 1980s are the neverending shifts in the public service organisational environment. No longer is welfare rights practice the preserve of local authority social services departments (if it ever was), but as public service boundaries become blurred with staff providing care services working alongside people from other professional backgrounds and employing bodies, welfare rights practice needs to be demystified so that a wider range of professionals can engage with it and understand how, at the right levels, it is a relevant part of their own professional practice and senior managers in partner organisations are helped to understand this.

A particular challenge lies in the fragmentation of local authority social services and social work departments as they are broken up into specialist services for children, adults and others. Where should welfare rights specialists 'belong' and how far is welfare rights practice viewed as relevant in these new organisations with their new modern 'missions'?

Of course it might be viewed as cynical to remind readers that history shows that the fragmentation of care services into multidisciplinary specialisms first ended with the Local Authority Social Services Act 1970 because it had been demonstrated that such bodies lacked economies of scale (among other things, making it more difficult to sustain specialisms such as welfare rights practice) and led to duplication of effort and people falling through the organisational gaps.

The political, social and economic environments, which modern welfare rights practice operates, pose significant challenges if welfare rights practice is to remain a unique and useful activity. Equally, there are numerous opportunities for welfare rights practice to continue to develop.

Welfare rights work has a proven track record and welfare rights services and practice have continued despite challenges and setbacks and, in many cases, they have flourished.

Chapters 3 and 4 will consider the actual practice of welfare rights work and the various methods of delivering it.

CHAPTER 3

EFFECTIVE WELFARE RIGHTS PRACTICE

OBJECTIVES

By the end of this chapter you should:

▦ Be able to consider the ethical basis of welfare rights practice

▦ Understand the practical application of welfare rights skills

▦ Be able to discuss advocacy skills.

THE ETHICAL BASIS OF WELFARE RIGHTS PRACTICE

This chapter considers some of the skills, ethics and practical aspects of welfare rights practice. However, it is not a technical guide to the legal aspects of benefit entitlement because there are other publications which serve this purpose and which are also regularly updated (please refer to Chapter 5).

Welfare rights practice is distinct because of its two main characteristics: the rights perspective and the 'instructional' relationship with the consumer. The rights- and advocacy-based nature of welfare rights practice largely arises because welfare rights problems are different from many other problems. These can be described as *bounded problems* – in other words, problems which are discrete, rule-based with a clearly identifiable problem and solution – as opposed to *unbounded problems*, which are more uncertain, are not governed by rules and which are often caught up with a contextual issue, for example interpersonal conflict (Watson and Watson 1986). An advocacy approach is not well suited to resolving an unbounded problem (it can actually make it worse) and an approach which is based on negotiation around mutually satisfactory objectives is more appropriate in such cases.

If we further analyse the two main characteristics of welfare rights practice, we can identify some key ethical principles which mark out welfare rights practice as a unique type of helping activity. These ethical principles also establish some standards for good practice – whether by welfare rights specialists or non-specialists.

The following principles behind welfare rights practice are derived from the rules of professional conduct for solicitors and are discussed at some length in Bateman (1996, 2000). They should be viewed as a whole and not seen in isolation from each other. The principles are as follows:

- Always act in the client's best interests
- Always act in accordance with the client's wishes and instructions
- Keep the client properly informed
- Carry out instructions with diligence and competence
- Act impartially and offer frank independent advice
- Maintain rules of confidentiality

ALWAYS ACT IN THE CLIENT'S BEST INTERESTS

This principle is a key one. It requires that welfare rights practice is focused on securing the maximum amount of benefit which the client is entitled to. It also means that the employing or host organisation must provide support and organisational space so that staff or volunteers can adhere to this principle. Indeed, the practitioner's ethical duty is to pursue this principle even if it risks causing conflict with the employer. The employer needs to be aware and accepting of the fact that such a principle will be followed.

ALWAYS ACT IN ACCORDANCE WITH THE CLIENT'S WISHES AND INSTRUCTIONS

Another key principle ensures that welfare rights work is based on the authority given by the client. It is a particularly empowering principle which aims to address the imbalance between advisers and consumers and seeks to ensure better accountability of welfare bureaucracies to their customers. Finally, it also sets down the basic ground rule for communications; the welfare rights advocate should not do anything which the client has not agreed to.

Of course, one must qualify the principle on the basis that it is the client's 'informed' wishes and instructions which matter. It is probably not legitimate to pursue a case which is completely unwinnable (e.g. an appeal against statutorily fixed benefit rates) or which would create a negative precedent for others – but some might debate this.

KEEP THE CLIENT PROPERLY INFORMED

This supports the second principle by ensuring that clients are aware of what is happening in their case and are able to make informed decisions about actions and advice. It also assumes that appropriate communication skills are used.

There are many practical ways to adhere to this principle. These include copying the client in to all letters, sharing drafts with the client before they are sent, making phone calls to the agency being advocated against while in the client's presence, having a policy of open access to case records and having a 'bring forward' system so that matters are reviewed at fixed periods. This also helps ensure that crucial deadlines are met.

CARRY OUT INSTRUCTIONS WITH DILIGENCE AND COMPETENCE

This principle aims to ensure that welfare rights advisers recognise and admit their limitations. It also implies that they know what they are talking about and have sought advice from an expert or they have used appropriate reference materials. If it is not possible to carry out the instructions with diligence and competence, the matter should be referred to someone else. This is not a sign of failure or incompetence; we all have our limits. This also illustrates the usefulness of all advisers identifying which level of advice they provide, that is Type I, II or II (see page 97), because it sets both boundaries and goals.

Inherent in this principle is the need to maintain and improve one's knowledge and skills and to build up knowledge of when and where to refer more complex matters to and to have agreed referral arrangements. There is strong evidence from practice that referrals which are effectively based on telling a service user where to go, fail. This is particularly for people coping with other pressures and issues or who simply feel powerless.

ACT IMPARTIALLY AND OFFER FRANK INDEPENDENT ADVICE

If the first four principles are about the style of welfare rights practice, this principle is concerned with implementing that style in practice. There is of course no such thing as 'impartial' advice in the sense that advice given about entitlements is neither value-free nor neutral and this is borne out in experience by comparing advice given by benefit officials and welfare rights advisers. The latter will frequently involve discussing tactics which might help someone to access a benefit or to challenge a decision; the style and flavour is very different. Impartial is meant in the sense of independent from the cause or organisation being advocated against.

Even how one completes a claim form and the presentation of supporting evidence to help a successful claim will be determined by the adviser's values, ethics and organisational loyalties.

It may well also be necessary to impart bad news or to have to offer advice in a context of realism such as, 'Your chances are borderline . . .'.

MAINTAIN RULES OF CONFIDENTIALITY

Trust between advocate and service users is vital. It is not that one wishes to hide any secrets nor to collude with anything illegal, but people using the service need to feel confident that they can divulge matters and these will not be passed on to the benefit authorities. In the same way, a business needs to know that its financial affairs will not be disclosed by its legal and accountancy advisers and that open conversations can take place with advisers secure in the knowledge that sound advice about the legality of a proposed course of action can be offered and debated.

Welfare rights problems are often associated with all manner of intimate and complex personal issues – from ill health to the details of personal relationships. To disclose these without permission would damage the trust and might even lead to a formal complaint.

In cases where the worker becomes aware of information which involves a risk to a third party (particularly if that third party is a child or is vulnerable or less powerful), the duty to protect that third party overrides a duty of confidentiality. Normally one agrees the ground rules for confidentiality with service users and this is a common exception found in policies of advice agencies.

An additional dimension to confidentiality has been added by the Data Protection Act 1998, which lays down eight data protection principles. These require that personal data about individuals must be kept secure, not passed on without the individual's permission (though there are significant exceptions associated with crime, health, education and social work) and the Act also grants people a right to see their personal data. This includes access to notes, emails, reports and photographs of them and highlights the need for effective confidentiality practices as well as opening up useful opportunities for welfare rights advocates to obtain information on behalf of claimants from benefit authorities (Information Commissioner 2001). The Freedom of Information Act 2000 has also opened up great opportunities for obtaining internal public body procedural policy and other information of a non-personal nature which can be very useful for understanding what the other side should or did do.

PRACTICAL WELFARE RIGHTS PRACTICE

Welfare rights practice can often be straightforward and it is also possible for non-welfare rights specialists to include it in their day-to-day work. To achieve this, experience shows that remembering a few key points is helpful. These have been summarised by Bateman and Somerville (2004) as follows:

> There are a number of effective approaches to welfare rights work. These approaches can reduce the frustration of dealing with often remote bureaucracies . . .
>
> Some things to remember:

- Always personally check the correct rules and interpretation . . .
- Keep up to date by reading, having up-to-date reference books, and attending training
- Build up a network of experts whom you can call on for help and support. Don't be embarrassed to call on them for advice – none of us know it all
- View welfare rights problems as inter-related and avoid tackling issues in isolation from one another
- Try to carry out a check of all benefit entitlement as a routine part of any assessment or when a financial issue is presented. There may be underclaiming of a benefit which doesn't spring to mind and which could thus solve a problem
- Avoid negotiating by phone and it's best to confirm things in writing
- Don't get overwhelmed by what seem to be impossible problems – all problems have some kind of solution and you may need just a small amount of help to find it
- The social security system uses National Insurance Numbers (NINOs) to identify benefit claimants. People without a NINO can be helped to apply for them and should receive a payment on account of their benefit while they wait for a NINO. Keep a record of NINOs and include them in communications with the Department for Work and Pensions, local authorities and HM Revenue and Customs.
- Gather supporting evidence for any argument from a variety of sources and present it in a way which supports the best rights interpretation
- It is often well worth the time to fill in claim forms – particularly for disability living allowance and attendance allowance. Even the best of us can find forms daunting to fill if unaided, let alone if you're experiencing poor self-esteem, turmoil, stress or any ill health or if English is not your first language
- Keep your interviewing skills sharpened and record important and useful facts that might have a bearing on benefit entitlement
- Build up your assertiveness skills

- Develop skills in researching a case and finding the most favourable argument
- Remember the power of rights which are enforceable by appeals and don't shy away from using these
- Never fib in order to try to get round benefit rules, but honestly present the facts in the best light. Never help people with completing a form, letter or phone call which includes facts that you know are untrue. If in any doubt, seek independent advice
- Seek specialist help in any fraud cases or if you suspect a service user is participating in fraudulent activity. With the latter, advise them of their duty to report relevant information to the benefit authorities and record that you have given this advice, even if they choose not to take it – in which case you have the option to not assist them.

(Bateman and Somerville 2004: 1)

Whether or not you are a specialist, you cannot go far wrong in welfare rights practice if you act in accordance with these while also operating within the ethical principles.

Provided that there is good access to a second tier welfare rights support service (which would provide training, consultancy and specialist casework help in more complex situations), non-specialists can successfully incorporate welfare rights work into their daily practice in a variety of ways without having to be experts and without a high risk of error. Depending on the organisational settings, the following are achievable and make a real difference to the lives of service users:

- undertaking a general benefits check as part of assessments of need
- responding to benefit and debt enquiries raised by service users, particularly to tackle less complex benefits problems
- including benefit maximisation and trouble-shooting as part of routine work on recovery of fines, rent and local tax debts
- considering the benefit implications of key life changes such as having a baby, adopting or fostering a child, a child or young person entering or leaving the care system, acquiring or parting with a partner, experiencing a bereavement, moving home, entering a care home or hospital, taking on a job or training, entering education, etc.
- using a benefits maximisation approach as part of any local authority obligation to provide financial support.

The following case study is an example of relatively uncomplicated welfare rights advice. It would have been possible for this to have been undertaken earlier in the chain of events (thus saving time and cost for the tenant and landlord alike) if the housing officer saw such work as part of her role and if she had had some training, information and other support to enable her to do this or even if she had sufficient basic knowledge to be put on inquiry that there may have been possible benefits issues here.

**BOX 3.1: CASE STUDY:
SAVING A FAMILY'S HOME**

Mrs Smith is aged 67. She is a local authority tenant who receives pension credit, housing benefit and council tax benefit. She has several health problems but has not claimed any benefits for these. Her adult son and daughter live with her. Her son works in a low paid job and her daughter is unemployed. Because her adult offspring live with her, she has a reduction in her housing benefit, but they are unable to make up the shortfall. As a result the family now have significant rent arrears and are facing possession action by their landlord.

The local authority housing officer who deals with their case asks them to make an offer to repay their rent arrears but does not carry out a benefits check because she does not think that welfare rights work is part of her remit. They agree a repayment arrangement but this is not adhered to, so the case proceeds to court.

Before the court hearing the family seek advice from a welfare rights adviser. Within ten minutes the adviser identifies that Mrs Smith could qualify for attendance allowance because of her health problems. This would be paid on top of her other benefits. Her daughter, who is her main carer, could claim carer's allowance and because she has no other income, would qualify for a higher amount of income support as a carer. In the circumstances, the family also might qualify for a retrospective discretionary housing payment (possibly for a short period) to help lessen, or even remove, the reduction in their housing benefit. In addition, the rent arrears can be paid by deductions from Mrs Smith's pension credit – not only at a lower rate than the 'realistic' offer agreed with the housing officer, but also without the inconvenience of having to travel to make the payments at the local housing office. The welfare rights adviser helped them to make claims for all these benefits.

This case study (based on true events) illustrates how straightforward income maximisation saved the family's home.

ADVOCACY

Advocacy is central to welfare rights practice and is one if its unique features. By 'advocacy' I mean the process of speaking up on behalf of another person (the client/customer/service user/etc.) and effective advocacy skills make a real difference to the success rate of welfare rights practice. It is this advocacy role which drives the ethical principles I have discussed earlier.

The role of advocate has long-standing acceptance within the nursing, medical and social care professions as well as among lawyers and advice workers and this is reflected in the various codes of professional practice and conduct. Advocacy by non-specialists is summarised by Payne as seeking 'to represent the interests of powerless clients to powerful individuals and social structures' (Payne 1997: 266).

Advocacy skills are a clearly defined set of skills which operate within the boundaries of the ethical principles which were discussed earlier in this chapter.

These skills include:

- Interviewing skills and evidence gathering skills – the best ways to collect information during a one-to-one interaction.
- Assertiveness – the ability to make one's position clear.
- Force – it may be necessary to use a more forceful approach (such as the willingness and stated desire to take matters further) and to have it in reserve.
- Legal knowledge and research – there is no substitute for knowing what you are talking about but no one knows it all. There are specific skills in researching legislation and caselaw and applying these to the best effect for the client.
- Keeping up-to-date.
- Negotiation – this is not about compromising but about achieving the best result for the client.
- Self-management – it is vital to organise oneself and to manage the time which is available so that crucial deadlines are achieved.
- Representation and litigation – it is often necessary to litigate something – take the dispute to a tribunal or some other formal arena. This ensures not only that a right becomes enforceable but also that one has a hearing before an impartial adjudicator rather than trying fruitlessly to persuade a benefits administrator of the flaws in their decision. The skills here are not just technical but knowing how to present the best case for a client in the most persuasive way.

(adapted from Bateman 2000)

INTERVIEWING SKILLS

The skills in obtaining accurate information from a service user, and to do so at the client's pace, are common to many types of activity. Because advocacy involves establishing facts or obtaining evidence, the sub-skills involved in listening, questioning (i.e. appropriate and selective use of direct and indirect questions) and observing non-verbal communication are key elements of interviewing skills.

It is of course essential that the client is at ease during any communication and is able to talk about the intimate personal details which are frequently involved in welfare rights problems. This may mean that several interviews are needed; rather than sitting down and working through a benefit application form, it may be necessary to start by having a conversation about a problem, asking the client to describe their perceptions and what they feel are the relevant facts.

It should go without saying that good quality facilities are also important – visually pleasing, spacious and soundproof interviewing rooms or offices make a huge difference and yet this is so often an area where costs are pared back and physical facilities in agencies which are on the claimant's 'side' are not infrequently worse than those found in social security offices.

Another area where costs may be skimped is on interpreters. While interpreting services do cost money and may take additional time and effort to access, they are essential for people whose first language is not English (including people whose main language is British Sign Language). Indeed, the frequent failure by the DWP to use interpreters is a cause of additional welfare rights work. Telephone-based interpreting services are not ideal and work best only for short-term or emergency communication.

Alongside interviewing is the process of gathering facts relevant to the issue. Benefits administration services are a key source of such information and should normally provide this provided that the customer has given their written consent. An alternative tactic is to ask, using data protection legislation, for all the information that an organisation holds about an individual.

It may also be necessary to interview carers about the customer's situation and needs, to approach relevant health, educational and social care practitioners who are also involved with the customer for information that they hold. However, relationships with such allies can easily become strained by requests for unnecessary information or which involves them in significant extra work. This is a particular issue with general practitioners and the level of requests for information from welfare rights advisers has arisen prompting discussion between the British Medical Association and central government. Part of the difficulty concerns the position of GPs as independent commercial contractors within a state run health service. Experience suggests that making very specific requests (perhaps with a pro-forma) is more likely to be cooperated with than a generalised request for information, perhaps sent off early on in the life of a case. GPs are entitled to charge for information in connection with benefit appeals, but not for information in connection with claims. If there is a pattern of charges being made for providing supporting medical evidence, it may be resolved by careful negotiation with local representative and primary care bodies as well as clarification about how and when information will be sought. Pointing out the health improvements associated with income maximisation and the reduction in stress from resolving benefit disputes may also help.

An associated task in the early stages of an advocacy task is gathering facts and information. This can include information from the benefits and tax credit authorities about how they have reached a decision and in the case of debts, copies of credit agreements, accounts and current stage of recovery action. The *Debt Advice Handbook* contains excellent guidance on how to handle this stage in debt advice cases (Madge *et al.* 2004).

EVIDENCE GATHERING SKILLS

Any activity which involves advising about the law, including welfare rights practice, is based on establishing important facts, obtaining evidence for these and then seeing how these support a particular interpretation about entitlement. A corollary of this is that one might explore an area of benefit entitlement (such as, 'Am I entitled to benefit X?') and then look for facts in a client's circumstances which support the entitlement.

Similarly one might be looking for evidence to challenge a refusal to pay a particular benefit – a very common activity because such a high proportion of benefit refusals and sanctions are based on poor quality factual information and frequently one just has to set out the facts in a clear manner to overturn a case.

However, such is the organisational culture within most DWP offices, which often presents as a combination of overwork, insularity and suspicion about claimants' honesty, the experience of welfare rights advisers is that they can find that it is very difficult to get even obviously wrong decisions reversed using the revisions and super-sessions procedures and have to appeal to a tribunal. This is an incredible waste of time and money for everyone not to mention the stress and hardship for claimants. This was borne out in a national survey of welfare rights advisers by the DWP's Standards Committee in 2004.

The types of factual information which is needed will vary from benefit to benefit and from person to person. Building up a wide factual picture (even of facts which do not appear at first to be relevant) can be useful as this can lead you to solutions which lie beyond the immediate problem – for example, a problem with housing benefit and the maximum amount allowed towards someone's rent may be solved by making a successful claim for a discretionary housing payment relying on a claimant's wider circumstances. Facts are likely to include the following:

*   Basic personal details, family composition, relationships, housing status, dates of birth, immigration and residence status, whether children are in full-time education and National Insurance numbers.
*   Housing costs – capital outstanding on mortgage and loans for repairs and improvements, rent (including details of any services included in the rent such as water, fuel or landlord services), annual council tax bill and council tax band.
*   Health – nature of any disability or health problems of the claimant and the people they claim for and, most importantly, the effects of this on their day-to-day activities and the prognosis and whether or not their condition has changed, plus an awareness of how they score against the personal capability assessment for incapacity benefit if they are under 60.
*   Details of any benefit or tax credit overpayments, how these arose, how they have been calculated, whether there are any benefits to be offset what the claimant did or didn't do and what did or didn't cause them.
*   Details of debts, who is owed what and what for, the legal status of credit and debts and details of any recovery action and what stage it is at.
*   Employment details including hours of work of claimant and any partner, gross and net earnings, costs associated with taking work, information about how earnings vary and details of previous tax year's income.
*   Childcare costs: hours and costs per week, whether childcare provider is registered or otherwise creates entitlement to help via tax credits, whether or not the hours and cost vary and number of children for whom childcare is paid.
*   Sufficient information about how benefits and tax credits have been assessed. This is partly a matter of experience but even very experienced advisers can find that amounts received each week are difficult to reconcile with assessments of

entitlement (for example, if someone has a mortgage or if they have deductions from their benefits to pay debts) and it is far from unknown for benefit administrators to make basic errors. It is possible to be sent a full written explanation of how a benefit or tax credit award has been calculated.

Alongside collecting such information, it is also useful to complete a standard written consent form so you can be given information by benefit authorities. If you work for an organisation, the consent should be granted to the organisation's staff to enable others to also help or provide cover if you are absent. The issue of consent is often a tiresome problem with the DWP in particular, as many staff do not adequately understand the legal basis of consent giving. The HM Revenue and Customs also insist on a very formalised approach to consent giving which can be a barrier for advisers. These problems partly lie in their staff turnover and recruitment of new staff who are confused about protocols for releasing information but also, it must be said, by some staff trying to obstruct access by third parties who may challenge and/or create extra work for them. There also seems to be an unfortunate habit in some parts of the DWP, HM Revenue and Customs and in some housing benefit services of losing consent forms or not adequately transferring the consent onto computerised records.

Collecting factual information should ideally take place early on in the process of an issue (though inevitably, additional or clearer facts may be needed at any time). This is because of the need to build up a full picture so that a proper benefits assessment can be done. It also reflects the stages of advocacy which characterise effective case advocacy. These were discussed in Bateman (1996, 2000) and comprise:

- presentation of the problem
- information gathering
- legal research
- interpretation and feedback
- active negotiation and advocacy
- litigation.

These stages can be identified in any piece of welfare rights practice and it is failure to work through each stage and move on to the next which often explains why welfare rights advocacy can fail.

ACTIVITY 3.1

Using a recent piece of welfare rights practice you have undertaken, identify the stages of advocacy in it. If the matter was referred on to a more experienced adviser, can you identify the latter stages in their work?

If the advocacy was not successful, were there any deficiencies in the earlier stages which contributed to this?

ASSERTIVENESS

It is impossible to act as an advocate if you are not assertive on behalf of the client. Assertiveness involves acting in a clear, direct and honest way and getting over the key points to the body one is advocating against. Assertiveness also includes the willingness and ability to take a problem up through the right appeal mechanisms and to use complaints and liaison procedures to challenge poor practice and wider service problems. Part of this may include being clear with the agency you are advocating against that failure to award the benefit being claimed at a particular stage will include the advocate making use of the next channel of appeal. The threat to appeal a social security problem to a tribunal has little effect on most benefit officials (though some housing benefit and homelessness staff will take heed because of the additional work involved in processing an appeal), but being clear that a matter might be taken to court or involve a complaint to an Ombudsman is often more effective.

Another remedy is to use publicity to highlight bad service: this tactic goes beyond just the usual appellate provisions but has been proven to be a highly effective way of enforcing people's rights and for challenging patterns of unlawful or unacceptable service.

Having confidence in one's abilities and in knowing what one is talking about is an important element of assertiveness and a well reasoned argument backed up by a clear understanding of the facts and accurate legal references feeds a cycle of confidence, assertiveness and successful outcomes.

FORCE

Going beyond mere assertiveness is the appropriate use of force. All welfare bureaucracies use forceful methods to protect their interests – denial of benefits, refusal to provide housing, threatening action on unpaid debts, recovery of overpayments, etc. They do not shirk from sending formal letters warning customers about the dire consequences if they do not do what is demanded. So the use of force is a legitimate tactic in welfare rights practice to protect clients – for example, legal action to ensure correct benefits are paid, against refusal of help or something which the customer appears to be entitled to or to defend a position.

The use of force may sometimes put advocates in a difficult position if they work for public sector bodies; there are numerous instances of social workers and welfare rights advisers within local authorities being told to 'tone down' their advocacy in the name of inter-agency cooperation. This is proving to be more of a problem in those local authorities which have developed joint teams with the DWP. However, it is also not unknown for complaints about forceful advocacy to be used as a rationale for ending or reducing local authority grants to advice services in the voluntary sector and it is not unknown for voluntary sector welfare rights and debt advisers to 'self-censor' their criticism and advocacy against any funders such as local authorities, which may also be guilty of poor practice in benefits administration, debt collection or housing rights.

Such problems can be resolved by clear and honest discussion about the importance of advocacy in ensuring pluralism and improved access to services, the consequent role of advocates and the wider legitimate function for staff in caring roles to act as advocates. It also requires bodies such as housing providers and the DWP to depersonalise matters and develop a more mature approach to advocacy and to recognise that it is not only a sign of a healthy democracy but also a way of identifying areas for improvement.

Force can sometimes involve the use of a bluff – but only when you are also certain that you can use whatever it is you are threatening. For example, in a rent arrears case where I was representing a tenant of a large commercial landlord in possession proceedings for rent arrears, the landlord's solicitor had added significant (but allowable and realistic) legal costs to their claim. I expressed surprise and said to the solicitor that I thought the costs were excessive and I was minded to challenge them. After short discussion with his client, the solicitor dramatically altered the costs claim, which was greatly advantageous to the tenant. This was just as well because if I had been forced to mount a challenge to the costs, I would not have known how to do it nor able at the time to find someone willing and able to do so. The bluff worked.

LEGAL KNOWLEDGE AND RESEARCH

Knowing what you are talking about and having a sound and up-to-date knowledge of the law on social security is vital. However, this is not to say that advocates with lesser skill and knowledge levels cannot do an effective piece of welfare rights practice – the solution is knowing what your limits are and having effective referral and consultation systems. How you can build and maintain a good knowledge base is discussed further on in this section but it is important to state that one cannot have too many welfare rights books; frequently the situation in many helping agencies is the reverse with perhaps one outdated welfare rights textbook available between a dozen staff. This can sometimes also be the situation in solicitor's firms and I've come across it in some smaller advice agencies. My all-time record was finding a book which was 12 years out-of-date in a social work team's bookcase.

This is a shortsighted approach which adds to the perception that welfare rights practice is time consuming and too complicated for non-experts. The majority of welfare rights problems can be resolved by using one of the standard welfare rights textbooks (see Chapter 5) and simply having ready access to an up-to-date book will pay for itself the first time it is used successfully. The Internet is a supplementary (but not a substitute) source of advice and information. And there are a number of useful on-line benefit calculators. Of course avoid overreliance on official sites such as those of the DWP or HM Revenue and Customs. Some sites (such as www.rightsnet.org.uk) have discussion boards where you can post questions for welfare rights advisers.

A large amount of welfare rights advice, particularly the less complex sort, is correcting basic mistakes by benefit providers – either factual errors or simple legal errors or in correcting a customer's own basic misunderstandings about benefit rules. Having a good basic knowledge of the rules of entitlement and then using a standard textbook or the Internet to find the answer can normally successfully resolve these problems.

At more sophisticated levels – for example, borderline cases and in appeals to tribunals – one has to apply a correspondingly more sophisticated legal approach. This involves use of the actual legislation and caselaw, applying rules of legal interpretation and finding either an interpretation or similar fact cases which support your arguments. The skills involved in this go beyond the scope of this book but were discussed in Bateman (1996, 2000) and the skills are also considered and explained in standard texts on legal method and legal interpretation.

The basic standard textbooks can be used in conjunction with each other; coverage of details and interpretation can vary from book to book and they will usually have footnotes which cite legal authorities for the main text. Use of these footnotes enables the adviser to quote actual legislation and caselaw and also internal DWP and HM Revenue and Customs guidance to support a particular argument or to point out an obvious mistake. Increasing amounts of internal guidance is now available on-line and that which is not can usually be obtained by making a formal request for its release under the Freedom of Information Act 2000 and the equivalent Scots and Northern Irish legislation.

BOX 3.2:   CASE STUDY: USING THE LAW

Mohan is aged 78. He has had a stroke which has left him seriously paralysed down his left side and unable to do many of the everyday tasks which he could previously do with no difficulty; he now needs help with things such as dressing, washing and bathing, cutting up food and getting around. He has been advised by the clinicians caring for him that he has recovered as much as he can be expected to. With help from his social worker he applies for attendance allowance. He receives a letter back advising him that he will be awarded the lower rate of the allowance after he has met the conditions of entitlement for six months – the date being six months after he had claimed the allowance. His claim had been made three months after he had his stroke.

His social worker consults a standard textbook and establishes that S65 Social Security Contributions and Benefits Act 1992 states that the six month period includes a period where someone has continually satisfied or is likely to have satisfied the disability conditions for six months. Therefore, the award of the allowance should start three months after his claim – i.e. six months after the stroke.

The social worker confirms the precise date of the stroke and writes a letter asking the DWP to revise its decision because of this error; this request is agreed to and the award is brought forward to the appropriate date. There is no other aspect of the claim which is in dispute.

continued

> *Box 3.2 con't.*
>
> Such scenarios are not uncommon and the adviser may not think of them in terms of evidence gathering and using the law. The solution clearly lies in researching and using the law to protect the service user's interests.

As well as textbooks, it is possible to make use of other people's expertise in order to research the law and to develop arguments which the front line worker can then use. This is where a second tier welfare rights service is particularly helpful and it is one of the most effective ways for a social work or other service to use its welfare rights resources and it can be particularly empowering and efficient. There are also national and regional second tier services, some of which (in England and Wales) are funded by the Legal Services Commission, which provide advice to advice workers and/or to generalists such as social workers and housing staff.

The Internet contains a growing amount of information and a list of useful websites is contained in Chapter 5. On-line resources have the advantage of being relatively easy to search and are available at little or no cost. However, there are currently no substitutes on-line for good textbooks and websites are not yet able to interpret the law and make informed judgments; indeed, such services may require a new form of information and communications technology to be developed.

KEEPING UP-TO-DATE

The social security system is constantly changing. Hardly a week goes by without something being changed – either a new piece of caselaw which changes some minor aspect of interpretation or new legislation to tidy up or adjust some rule or other. As well as these everyday changes, there are the larger changes brought about by more radical shifts in government policy such as the changes in 1988 (considered in Chapter 1) and the introduction of tax credits and pension credit in 2003. Keeping on top of all this is a real challenge for any welfare rights adviser and, if inadequately supported, it can be really difficult for a non-specialist. There are ways to manage this, however, and it goes back to the level of competence expected of the adviser – be they an expert or otherwise.

For non-specialists, participation in the following could be an appropriate model of updating which fits with the suggested typology on page 97 and which is used by several local authorities:

- one-day, annual updating courses covering major changes in the benefits system (which may not be required every year)
- four-monthly briefings of about two hours by welfare rights advisers covering recent changes and anticipated developments
- an administrative process to ensure that welfare rights reference books are ordered annually

- a regular four-page bulletin written by welfare rights advisers summarising key changes and issues.

However, none of the above will really work unless there is adequate investment in the basics – enough books, adequate access to a helpline for advice and referral to staff and above all some foundation training.

Foundation training is often skimped – organisations are wary of releasing staff and incurring costs of paying for courses and frequently managers who commission training make requests such as, 'Please can you do a one-day course which covers the benefits system'. Experience shows that this is not possible and has been less possible since the introduction of tax credits. A basic course to cover the ground to enable people to apply first aid advice, identify general unclaimed benefits and to make informed referrals takes about 20 hours, ideally with some element of assessed work. Beyond this, one should also consider providing more specialised one-day courses such as benefits for people with particular disabilities, benefits for young people, how to tackle housing benefit problems, benefits and social care charges, understanding debt and about how to challenge benefit refusals. There is an active and diverse market of individuals and organisations offering welfare rights training, much of it aimed at non-specialists.

Levels of welfare rights training across the public sector vary greatly. Some organisations see it as an important area and have made a commitment to invest and to ensure that staff are well resourced. Others just do not see it as their 'problem', hoping that this organisational denial will mean that the problem goes away. Even among bodies which do invest in welfare rights training and support, the training element is often approached on a voluntary basis, and as a result the more interested and motivated staff will attend courses. This makes for another problem; the more engaged and therefore better informed members of staff can feel imposed upon and resentful towards colleagues who avoid welfare rights practice. It also means that the standard of service that a customer receives depends on the personal interests and values of an individual member of staff: this is not a rational way to provide any service. As with any other area of activity, it is therefore crucial that there is an unambiguous commitment by senior managers to develop welfare rights practice and an explicit expectation about the level of welfare rights practice which staff are expected to engage in.

Despite improvements since the 1990s, often little time is devoted to welfare rights teaching on professional social work training courses. Some institutions appear to try and 'cover the lot' in a couple of hours, perhaps by calling in a local welfare rights adviser. Others treat it as an integral part of the curriculum and accord it the same status as other areas of practice training and have assessed work (the latter is probably a crucial element in getting welfare rights practice taken seriously).

Those organisations which have invested in welfare rights services to empower and support staff to engage in practice have found that it does work and the results are there to see. Problems with staff making mistakes or getting out of their depth usually arise in those organisations which allow staff to dabble in it and throw the occasional bit of training at it with little or no other support.

The updating needs of welfare rights specialists are also important. The require-ments of various quality systems (such as the Community Legal Service Quality Mark), which welfare rights advisers in England and Wales will normally hold, mean that at a minimum their employing organisation must have systems in place for updating. The level of investment in training and development needs to be such that staff can comply with this requirement and can then advise competently about the complex issues which they are presented with.

This means that welfare rights advisers probably need to consider an initial investment in their training (depending on previous experience) of about 60 hours within the first year of practice. Thereafter, as well as having adequate resources to buy the specialist texts in Chapter 5, the following are normally viewed as essential:

- attending more in-depth courses and seminars – 25 hours a year is probably an achievable minimum, the Community Legal Service Specialist Level Quality Mark currently requires just 6 hours
- membership of and attendance at meetings of the National Association of Welfare Rights Advisers and regional and local groups where these exist
- subscriptions to the following journals: *The Adviser* (Shelter and National Association of Citizens Advice Bureaux), *Welfare Rights Bulletin* (published by Child Poverty Action Group), *Touchbase* (DWP), *Legal Action* (Legal Action Group), *Disability Rights Bulletin* (Disability Alliance)
- a system for daily updating: the website www.rightsnet.org.uk provides a ready system for such updating activity and time spent checking it is time well spent
- access to other specialists for help and support, particularly on complex or ambiguous issues.

Additional resources will be required for those who also provide debt and/or housing advice.

In addition, for both specialists and non-specialists, inclusion of welfare rights training and developmental needs should figure in processes such as training needs analyses, annual appraisal/performance reviews, supervision and mentoring activities.

NEGOTIATION

Negotiation is the process of reaching agreement and is particularly useful in welfare rights practice when a case is weak or the remedies to enforce a right are not useable. That said, the customer is less powerful than the large welfare bureaucracies and the core nature of a welfare rights problems – the denial of legally guaranteed rights, means that the bargaining and trading of positions and concessions during negotiation can easily leave the client at a disadvantage – though I have occasionally come across local authority benefit officials suggesting it as an alternative to giving full entitle-ment (which is clearly an unacceptable approach for a welfare rights practitioner to cooperate with). Negotiation is not an alternative to use of the appeals procedures or of the statutory provisions for seeking a revision or supersession in social security.

However, in borderline cases particularly, the principles behind good negotiation can be helpful.

Negotiation is also appropriate when trying to press for improvements in benefits services or for local benefit providers to change practices or their interpretation. Examples would be less intrusive questioning by benefit providers of young people making claims and accepting that people with mental health problems who attend day care services should be exempted from the personal capability assessment. However, such negotiations take place done within the parameters of the law and broadly accepted interpretation (e.g. one could not agree to waive the capital limit for income support).

Negotiation is not about reaching a compromise – in itself an alien concept when dealing with a regulated system of entitlements, but about finding a solution for the customer which involves a step-change by the other side, preferably by enabling the other side to concede ground gracefully. Negotiation cannot (and should not in constitutional terms) enable a benefit provider to step outside the law – for example to allow someone who is clearly not entitled to benefit to be awarded it.

Negotiation can be used in welfare rights practice to help advocate for people to be awarded Social Fund community care grants or discretionary housing payments or at a strategic level, to achieve cooperation from benefit providers for take-up work, or for handling large volumes of appeals cases.

It might also be used in, for example, individual chronic rent arrears cases with an history of broken, reasonable repayment agreements, where legal arguments may be weak (though, even then one should be confident that are no 'technical' defences which could be mounted). The power that the negotiator has is the ability to enforce rights and to take a course of action which might involve costs to the other side. This places the welfare rights practitioner on a stronger footing if they are clear about it.

It is critical that one maintains that position of strength. This is partly because during negotiations each side will see the other as more powerful, so having a powerful stance to begin with is more likely to get better results for the customer.

The *Debt Advice Handbook* (Madge *et al.* 2004) contains several excellent pages about negotiation as a tactic and how to manage some of the responses one can receive, which can vary from outright hostility to attempts to manipulate. While primarily aimed at debt advice work, where problems can include unbounded ones, the approaches can also be relevant in welfare rights work provided that it is done in the context of the law affecting a particular case, particularly in cases involving exercise of discretion where facts are weak or with, for example, seeking to have an overpayment written off or reduced. Adopting approaches from standard texts on negotiation (such as Fisher and Ury 1981). Madge *et al.* (2004) suggest the following elements for successful negotiation and I have added some of my own comments:

- Separate the messenger from the message. Treat the other side with respect but not by trying to please them with offers (the latter is an approach which weakens your position).
- Avoid emotional involvement in the outcome. This can be difficult when dealing with a remote, obstinate, judgemental and incompetent benefits administration.

- Distinguish between aims and means. One may be able to get a result for the client which also happens to meet the needs of the other side. Again, this can and should be done without conceding ground.
- Recognise organisational constraints. In particular go up the hierarchy and identify who has the power to make decisions rather than engage in fruitless debates with junior front line employees. With benefits administrations, this quickly leads you to the conclusion that it is legitimate to involve politicians in the process.
- Search for mutual benefit and gain. 'If you agree to X, it saves you having to do Y'.
- Establish objective criteria. As well as trying to have objective outcomes, this can also attempt to steer unbounded problems into the bounded problem arena and the clearer remedies of an advocacy-based approach which characterise welfare rights practice.
- Allow irrational negotiators to have their say then overbid and compromise, appear to agree, set up a common enemy and offer to solve their problem if they adopt your approach. If necessary, repeat the arguments.

Madge *et al.* (2004) also suggest lines to take when faced with time-honoured arguments such as 'we are not a charity' or 'if we allow this, it will open the floodgates' (Madge *et al.* 2004: 19ff.).

It is important to try to reflect negotiations either in writing or at least by confirming agreements in writing. Welfare rights practice is riddled with instances of discussions with benefits officials over the phone which are then subsequently lost, denied as ever having happened because there is no record, overruled or occasionally even lied about. I would suggest that even routine discussions about how a case has been decided are confirmed in writing so there is a record and the benefits provider also then knows that you are acting for the client and written communication reduces the scope for emotion to distract from judgement. Often it can be difficult to talk to decision makers in the DWP – possibly a deliberately obstructive strategy among more junior staff, and a letter setting out an argument will (one hopes) get to the right person. A series of letters can also form a useful audit trail – particularly useful for quality standards and for handling any complaint from a customer.

Telephone conversations are also a less structured form of communication, requiring innate and quick responses, both of which undermine the calm, unemotional and logical processes needed for effective advocacy and negotiation. As one will also often be talking to fairly junior operatives in a social security bureaucracy, this means that doing it by phone is not the best way – a particular problem because government is increasingly insisting on channelling increasing amounts of social security customer service by telephone. But then there is always email.

Finally, one disadvantage of the written medium is that letters can and do get lost within benefit bureaucracies and there can often be a delay in getting a reply. This is why a diary system to follow up communications is important, as is an adequate case record showing actions taken. It is stating the obvious that it is essential to keep copies of letters.

SELF-MANAGEMENT

Any activity requires effective self-management coordination. Welfare rights work particularly requires it because there are significant deadlines for getting things done. For example, there are time limits for making an appeal or even seeking an explanation of why a negative decision has been made. Failure to adhere to deadlines can have severe consequences for the service user and many promising cases fail because advisers have been unaware, overlooked or muddled about a key deadline for action on an issue.

Self-management includes a range of skills – time management, written skills, creative thinking, decision making and stress management. To enable these to happen – particularly when applying skills associated with files and documents associated with welfare rights practice – it is important to have procedures and processes in place to support practitioners to be effective self-managers. The Community Legal Service Quality Mark (discussed on page 107), is particularly designed to ensure that advisers have systems for file management, bring-forward dates, etc.

Further discussion about self-management techniques in welfare rights practice can be found in Bateman (2000).

REPRESENTATION AND LITIGATION

Representing a service user before a tribunal or some other forum is the pinnacle of welfare rights practice and one which has proven results. The ability to take a dispute to an independent tribunal and to have the opportunity to make your case with or without skilled representation acts as a valuable check on the power of the social security bureaucracy and is an effective way to challenge negative benefit decisions and there are some issues which have a staggeringly high success rate – for example, appeals against refusals of incapacity benefit. As such it is an important feature of a democratic society.

Any form of litigation also opens up the potential for using it to push back the boundaries of entitlement, via test cases.

While the original aim of tribunals was to provide an accessible form of justice which did not require skilled representation, having a representative does and always has made a huge difference to success rates. The ever growing complexity of social security law also means that as far as possible appellants should always be represented and representation is not a task to be undertaken lightly.

The statistics about appeal outcomes illustrate both the scale of appeals and the difference that representation makes – which is why it is strange that the government has taken the view recently that people should not need representation. These ratios have remained fairly static over the years, even though the number of appeals has reduced because of falling working age claimant numbers and tighter rules about appeals introduced in 1999 (see Box 3.3).

BOX 3.3:   APPEAL STATISTICS FOR QUARTER ENDING 31 MARCH 2004

Success rate of appeals where the appellant has asked for an oral hearing	52.1%
Success rate of appeals where the appellant agreed to have the case decided on the papers rather than orally	21.0%

Success rates when appellant attends alone

Attendance allowance	48.6%
Disability living allowance	57.7%
Housing benefit	32.5%
Incapacity benefit (personal capability assessment)	61.8%
Income support	40.3%
Industrial injuries disablement benefit	46.5%

Success rates when appellant is represented and representative and claimant both attend

Attendance allowance	60.6%
Disability living allowance	68.0%
Housing benefit	62.5%
Incapacity benefit (personal capability assessment)	73.2%
Income support	67.8%
Industrial injuries disablement benefit	56.3%

Source: DWP (2004) *Work and Pensions Statistics 2004*. London: Department for Work and Pensions, pp. 213, 215 and 216.

Despite the success rate on appeals, it is still frustrating (and indicative of the DWP's introspective culture of denial) to hear government ministers repeating the line of their civil servants that as there are about 200,000 appeals a year out of several million benefit decisions, the success rate of appeals does not reflect badly on the DWP's overall level of performance. If the social security bureaucracy is so capable of getting it right, it is puzzling that a strand in government policy is to extend the range of issues which have no formal rights of appeal. For example, the new education maintenance allowances, decisions to defer or waive work-focused interviews, the Jobcentre Plus Personal Adviser's Fund, recovery of tax credit overpayments and the job grant.

The right to representation at social security tribunals is enshrined in law: Regulation 49(8) of the Social Security and Child Support (Decisions and Appeals) Regulations 1999 (with parallel rights for tax credits appeals) gives an appellant the right to be accompanied and represented by anyone of their choice. Over the years this right has been clarified by caselaw. In Commissioner's Decision CIB/2058/2004, it was held that representatives have a useful role in gathering evidence to help the tribunal reach a decision and that because 'good representation enhances the quality of the decision-making in a tribunal'(Commissioner Jacobs in CIB/2058/2004 para 14), they should be wary of not adjourning if a representative cannot attend. The Commissioner also stated:

> In 1989, Hazel and Yvette Genn wrote a Report for the Lord Chancellor on The Effectiveness of Representation at Tribunals. They concluded at page 247: 'The evidence presented in this report leads inescapably to the general conclusion that specialist representation at tribunals increases the likelihood that those who bring their cases before tribunals will succeed. . . .
>
> 'Unless the activities of representatives are thought to lead tribunals into allowing unmeritorious cases, the conclusion must be that representation increases the accuracy of tribunal decision-making. Representatives do this by furnishing tribunals with the information needed to reach reasoned decisions, based on all the relevant facts of the case, and on the law which relates to the case. In investigating cases, obtaining evidence, and advocating cases, representatives are ensuring that appellants whose cases have merit, are given the best chance of succeeding before the tribunal.'

The same Commissioner in a paper to the Social Security Law Practitioner's Association put forward a number of propositions about the conduct of representatives which he had distilled from Commissioner's Decisions. The propositions are that there are duties on representatives to

- have authority to act for the person who is appealing
- attend the hearing
- put the strongest arguable case for the client (while also not pursuing hopeless arguments)
- be polite
- obtain evidence on time

- adduce relevant oral evidence at the hearing
- work within the chairman's control of procedure at the hearing
- be honest to the tribunal.

The Commissioner concluded that tribunal representation had become increasingly skilled and professional and there is a case of regulation of representatives (Jacobs 2004).

It has also been held in caselaw that there is no absolute right to representation under the European Convention on Human Rights (CJSA/5101/2001) (though a string of cases shows that excluding or silencing a representative is not acceptable) that the bad conduct of a case by a representative can jeopardise a hearing (CDLA/1839/2000 para 7). The ability for local authority welfare rights representatives to represent in cases against their own local authority was discussed on page 3.

So undoubtedly, representation before appeal bodies has become more complex and, perhaps elitist, but there is still scope for non-experts to represent, and indeed, they are still a regular feature at tribunals. This is possible because of the duty on tribunals to act in an inquisitorial and less formal manner. However, I would generally recommend that non-expert representatives should attempt to obtain skilled help and representation with tribunal hearings if at all possible. However, in many places it is still not possible to obtain such help.

The skills involved in representation include the following:

- Involving the client – letting the client speak appropriately but briefing the client beforehand about what issues to mention and what to avoid, within the bounds of truthfulness. When a well-prepared client who is clear about the facts and arguments speaks, it can be highly persuasive. We have all had cases where a client has sprung damaging new evidence on the other side midway through a case or has needlessly upset carefully made plans. Good briefing and preparation reduce the chances of this happening. It is also important to seek to empower the client and not for the client's often great sense of disempowerment to be reinforced by someone else playing the expert and taking control. Equally, there are some clients who want and/or need just that.
- Carefully preparing the paperwork, including evidence and a written submission, setting out your arguments and citing legal authority for any propositions. The submission should be sent to the tribunal in good time before the hearing. Producing one at the hearing not only irritates the tribunal but also means that the client is disadvantaged by the tribunal possibly missing key points. Ideally a submission should contain a summary of the main facts and a summary of the appellant's case and what decisions the tribunal should reach, followed by more detailed arguments.
- Using rules of interpretation and rules of evidence (as these apply to tribunals), to challenge the other side's assertions and evidence.
- Obtaining and supplying evidence to contradict or weaken the other side's evidence.
- Making sure that all deadlines are adhered to and that those who have to attend the tribunal do so.

- Identifying and interviewing any witnesses and knowing what to ask and what not to ask them. Being clear why the witnesses are being called and what you want to get them to say. Then going on to question any witnesses in ways which are consistent with this.
- Testing out possible weaknesses in your arguments and evidence and having answers.
- Having skills in persuasion and talking – knowing when to stay silent, maintaining eye contact and tone of voice, presenting the case in a logical sequence which helps you take the tribunal where you want it to go, allowing pauses for the chairman to take notes. If you get nervous, use your right hand to hold your left wrist!

The right to litigate and appeal a welfare rights issue is hugely empowering for people who otherwise would have little option but to accept a decision which reduced their standard of living, which impoverished them or which might even have larger consequences. Ultimately it enables welfare rights practice to be taken seriously and to be able to make a difference.

The difference the law can make is epitomised by the test case strategy. This has long been a core part of welfare rights practice and over the years we can point to a string of successful legal challenges which have pushed back the barriers of entitlement and have resulted in more dignified treatment of claimants. Examples of test cases include:

- *Mallinson* – help with walking and reading qualify for disability living and attendance allowances
- *Collins* – paring back the effect of the habitual residence test on unemployed people
- *Nessa* – successfully challenging the DWP's accepted wisdom that only those in the UK for at least three months can get means-tested benefits
- *Fairey* – help with social activities qualifies for disability living and attendance allowances
- *Ex parte CPAG* – DWP cannot delay processing a benefit claim without limit of time
- *Bate* – severe disability premium for people who live in other's households
- *W v Secretary of State for Work and Pensions* – improved access for lone parents to help with mortgage costs
- Plus countless Social Security and Child Support Commissioner Decisions.

CHAPTER 4

DEVELOPING WELFARE RIGHTS PRACTICE

OBJECTIVES

By the end of this chapter you should:

▨ Be able to distinguish different types of welfare rights practice and delivery models

▨ Be able to discuss funding issues

▨ Understand the importance of quality and performance improvement

▨ Be able to build and sustain a welfare rights service.

EXAMPLES OF WELFARE RIGHTS PRACTICE

There is not a single model of welfare rights practice and the range of activities under the welfare rights banner varies according to local needs and priorities and the resources available as well as the organisational values of a particular agency.

In some areas there is little involvement by non-welfare rights specialists but in others, welfare rights services have successfully demonstrated how they can engage non-specialists in acting as a front line source of advice and referrals. In some areas there are large welfare rights services based in local authorities, complemented by a range of voluntary sector provision. In other areas, there may be one or two, or even (more commonly) none in a local authority and a sprinkling of provision in the voluntary sector. Whatever their size, specialist welfare rights services are all far smaller than the social security agencies – just one local social security office will have many more staff than even a large local welfare rights agency. This means that they frequently have to assess where their impact will be greatest.

There is a rich range of welfare rights activity which takes place in a variety of different settings. Examples include the following:

- Second tier welfare rights services within social services and social work departments to support non-specialist staff and to take complex referrals. There has also been a growth in welfare rights services based in housing associations (as discussed in Chapter 2). The strengths and weaknesses of first and second tier services are discussed at more length later in this chapter.
- Front line welfare rights advice services provided by or funded by local authorities and/or a variety of other funding – and juggling the different funding streams is creating its own problems.
- Front line services located within health care settings and which also provide some second tier services such as training to clinical staff.
- Welfare rights services delivered and funded via local Sure Start projects and aimed at parents using these services.
- Services (such as the Islington Schools Project) which target parents and carers via schools.
- Services aimed at people entering or re-entering the labour market after a long period of worklessness. Several services now exist independently from the DWP and occasionally work under contract to the DWP while retaining their autonomy.
- Services aimed at maximising incomes of those who use social service such as residential care and community care services. Some services are provided by voluntary bodies under contract to local authorities, others by a combination of local authority welfare rights advisers or finance staff who have been trained and supported by welfare rights advisers. The shortfalls of the models of joint DWP/local authority teams being promoted (or more accurately, continually nagged) to local authorities by the Pension Service are considered in Chapter 2.
- Specialist welfare rights staff (employed by both local authorities and voluntary bodies) targeting particular groups which experience difficulty accessing services, or who have additional needs or where there is evidence of significant under-claiming. These include services targeted at people who

    - have sensory impairments
    - are parents of children with a disability
    - are ex-offenders or families of prisoners
    - have rent or council tax debts
    - are HIV positive or who have AIDS
    - have long-term mental health needs
    - are young people leaving local authority care
    - have a learning disability
    - attend special schools
    - belong to black and minority ethnic groups

- have a terminal illness
- suffer from particular medical conditions (usually funded via charities for such conditions).

There is also a rich tapestry of benefit take-up work going on around the UK. Examples include:

- data-matching housing and council tax benefit records to identify unclaimed benefits (usually tax credits, income support or pension credit), targeting people identified by such activity with letters and/or visits to check their benefits and helping them claim the benefits they have missed out on
- using local authority and National Health Service registers of carers and children with disabilities to do similar work
- using general practitioners' patient records to target particular groups of known underclaimers or people with particular health problems
- contacting parents of pupils attending special schools and inviting them to come to the school for a benefits check by a welfare rights adviser
- doing similar work at day centres for both carers and service users
- targeting specific groups via faith organisations
- mailing and visiting people living in sheltered housing
- promoting large-scale take-up initiatives to wider groups of people on low incomes via local authority newspapers
- setting up advice desks when pensioners have their bus passes renewed
- targeting people living in residential care homes who are not supported by a local authority
- visiting every pensioner over the age of 85 in an area to do a benefits check.

MODELS OF DELIVERY

Given the diversity of welfare rights services, it is no surprise that there is not a standard model of service delivery. There two main types of service:

- front line or first tier services
- second tier services.

However, in practice, to some extent many services are hybrids of both types.

Front line or first tier services

As the name suggests, a front line service is advice activity provided directly by advisers to the public, whether by phone, email or face-to-face. This includes not just advice given by specialists but also advice provided by non-specialists. Ultimately, any welfare rights practice is meaningless unless it involves direct engagement with customers – and even second tier advice service frequently include an element of direct casework.

In recent years, there has been an emphasis on providing advice by media such as interactive television and Internet. Such approaches clearly should be part of any advice provision, but there are limitations. First, the quality of Internet-based advice varies tremendously and some services struggle to ensure that their web-based material is up-to-date. Second, no one has yet managed to develop software which can adequately cope with the complexity and interpretational aspects of this work (though the government is exploring the potential primarily as a way to reduce disputes – a questionable outcome). There are several computer programs which will calculate means-tested benefit entitlement; indeed, advice giving is best done with such a package because they are invaluable when calculating entitlement to multiple benefits and tax credits, but even these rely on the operator exercising some judgement about entitlement and interpretation of entitlement and they still need the adviser to actually interview the client. There are some packages where the service user can interact with the software, but these have had to be simplified so that only the more common and straightforward areas of entitlement are identified.

Of particular interest is the work within Citizens Advice Bureaux funded by government to enable advisers to directly access benefit records. This raises some questions about how far they can maintain both their actual and perceived independence (Treloar 2004) but it is likely that such direct access arrangements will be built on in future years and provided the rights safeguards are there, they could provide a speedier means of resolving straightforward problems (particularly correcting basic errors by DWP staff).

For welfare rights workers, there are also a number of computer software packages for recording advice on a client database and which also enable wider performance and policy information to be extracted and the ever falling price of computers means that funding IT developments is less of a challenge.

Of course, for customers themselves, there are also the limitations caused by the digital divide with the majority of low income households still being without computers and even some without a telephone.

Some welfare rights services offer direct telephone-based advice for the public and the Legal Services Commission is currently funding some services to provide such advice. Telephone-based advice has the advantage of being accessible for many and it is possible to deliver high volumes of work. The difficulty is that it is best suited to one-off queries where one can confidently provide advice to the caller and you know that they will be able to get a result on the basis of what they have been told. Even in one-off queries you cannot always be confident that your advice will be accepted by the benefit authorities and/or the caller will call back for help if they have a negative response when relying on your advice. Telephone-based advice usually becomes deficient when something which involves legal interpretation arises, if there is a dispute about entitlement or even with matters such as filling in a disability living allowance claim form (in itself not a neutral activity and one where questions of phraseology and interpretation arise). Then there are all those people who have difficulty accessing telephone-based advice – people with hearing problems, those whose first language is not English, people who cannot make calls in privacy and people who are worried about the cost of their phone bills.

A further problem with telephone-based advice which has been identified in advice agencies is that it is stressful for the call handlers – continually fielding enquiries is wearing, and adviser motivation and quality can easily suffer. The call centre response of using scripts (an approach loved by the DWP for its call centres) may help people to give the right corporate message but is a recipe for the lowest common denominator in advice work.

However, a telephone-based advice service is often used as an important back-up system for benefit take-up campaigns and inevitably the ability to provide good access means that telephone-based advice will continue to feature as a key part of advice work. The key will be to understand its strengths and weaknesses.

A major part of front line advice work is still carried out in face-to-face interviews. This has the advantage of providing much better quality communication, the ability for the enquirer to also show relevant papers to the adviser. Face-to-face advice work also means that trust between client and adviser is easier to establish.

Second tier services

Second tier advice services usually operate by providing advice and support to first tier or front line services. This includes offering consultancy for non-specialists by telephone and email, training, team briefings, newsletters and leaflets, policy work using case studies as evidence for arguing for changes in service by benefit providers and they usually also include a referral arrangement for complex cases with the second tier agency taking on the actual casework or doing so in tandem with the referrer as a skill development exercise.

Second tier work will also include running an information system so that the non-specialist staff are kept up-to-date with changes in benefits legislation (perhaps by regular briefings, a newsletter and/or email updates), publishing leaflets written from a customer-oriented rights perspective or aimed at particular customer groups, therefore filling gaps left by official leaflets.

The majority of welfare rights services within local authorities, and some external bodies funded by local authorities, operate as second tier services (or as hybrid services), and given the ever present limits on resources, developing a second tier welfare rights service has been found to be the best way to achieve maximum impact for the amount of money spent. It also engages others in welfare rights practice and can avoid the dumping syndrome.

Second tier services can be highly effective and indeed, one can argue they are a necessary part of any advice provision. Research confirms this:

> The evidence that second tier services add value to the work of first tier services is persuasive. The support provided by the second tier helps to raise the standards of first tier services, can increase their breadth and depth and ultimately, contribute to better outcomes for clients.
>
> (Steele and Searjant 1999)

A reasonable conclusion therefore is that one needs a mix of welfare rights service methodologies and delivery mechanisms in order to be effective. Locating all resources in one agency or adopting a policy of passing on every benefits problem will not reach even a small minority of the people who need to be reached.

ACTIVITY 4.1

What are the various strengths and weaknesses of first and second tier welfare rights services?

VOLUNTARY OR STATUTORY AGENCY?

One of the debates which occurs from time to time is whether welfare rights services should be placed within the local authority or within the voluntary sector. The argument is put that advisers who are based in the latter are independent and therefore better able to act as advocates and client centred advisers.

Experience shows that the independent sector may not always be as independent as some say – many of us have examples of voluntary advice agencies being 'leant on' by local authority funders for advocacy which is felt to be too vigorous, particularly when it involves advocacy against the funder. Similarly there are many instances of voluntary sector advice agencies limiting their advocacy because of the source of funding.

There is also some evidence that people from certain community groups tend to underuse voluntary sector advice agencies. For example, people from black and minority ethnic groups, young people and very elderly people tend to be under-represented in Citizens Advice Bureaux enquirer statistics. This may be due to wrongful perceptions about image or due to physical access problems, but whatever the cause, it will disenfranchise some people who need advice if there is not a plurality of organisations who are equipped to handle queries.

In response to such shortfalls in advice access, many black and minority ethnic voluntary bodies have developed advice services as an adjunct to their other services and one concern is that the increasingly professionalisation of advice work could further marginalise such underfunded and often small groups.

Experience also shows that welfare rights service within local authorities can act as effectively as advocates as those employed or volunteering within voluntary bodies. This is particularly true if they are based either within a social services setting or a corporate chief executive's department. It may be necessary to develop protocols around advocacy on any benefits or services administered by the local authority and supportive management which embraces the pluralism of welfare rights work and which respects the need for advocacy is essential.

Location of a welfare rights function inside a local authority also opens up many opportunities to address poverty. Indeed, welfare rights staff within local authorities have often been the champions of an anti-poverty perspective and have been able to positively influence many services – for example advising on criteria for school uniform grants, devising processes for improving take-up of free school meals, setting up benefit take-up systems within housing benefit services and developing corporate debt collection strategies which seek to maximise debtors' incomes and create realistic and sustainable repayment arrangements. There are also a number of technical welfare rights issues which are peculiar to local authority social services functions (for example, the effect of residential care on benefits and the effect of the childcare system on parents' benefits and tax credits). An in-house service will inevitably be much better placed to tackle these.

There is also the fact that some of our poorest and most vulnerable citizens are those who rely on local authority services. Location within social care services, in whatever shape they are configured, thus enables welfare rights advice and advocacy to be provided to people who often face huge issues in their lives and who may not be able to easily access external advice provision. It also means that anxieties about client confidentiality do not get in the way of referrals and for an organisational one-stop approach to be developed. Finally, a service located outside the local authority will always have greater difficulty influencing inside and in creating the synergy with local authority staff which enables effective and timely referrals to be made. And as Fimister stated: 'internal services can offer input to policy, publicity and staff training which can be much more problematic for outside bodies – especially the policy aspect' (Fimister 1986: 58).

A preferable model is what Fimister (1986) described as the 'mixed economy' of advice provision. This ensures a mix of provision provided through different outlets and organisations which helps ensure a better reach of advice provision. In many areas there are also successful models of collaboration such as bodies coming together under local umbrella groups to share experiences and expertise, to undertake joint work and to increase their impact by jointly lobbying and monitoring local benefit providers. And as long as local authorities have a hand in benefit provision, there will be a need for external bodies to scrutinise and challenge them on such issues, particularly if local authority staff have been 'advised' not to advocate vigorously on the issue.

Smaller organisations can face major problems delivering a high quality service because they do not have the same economies of scale as larger bodies. Not only are financial and staff time costs likely to be greater because of the overhead costs of an organisation such as insurance, audit, payroll and servicing the management committee, but also a very small staff group has less ability to provide adequate staff cover (in a small group it is not unknown for 25 to 50 per cent of the workforce to be absent if just one person is sick) and less ability to release people for training and development activities.

Larger providers, on the other hand, are better placed to cover temporary staff gaps, to release people for training, to organise their own training, to be able to buy specialised reference materials and to develop mini-specialisms among its workforce. In the 1970s one could operate by having two part-time advisers behind a table in a church hall using a couple of small textbooks (and some of us did effective work using such approaches). For better or worse, the present day advice agenda is infinitely more complex and such methods of delivery struggle to serve the customer well.

Small organisations may also operate in an area where other small organisations operate. This can make the tasks associated with commissioning, monitoring and coordinating services very difficult and complex for funders which discourages them from further investment. A compromise approach is for small advice bodies to pool certain overheads and to liaise with funders and commissioners via a single umbrella body.

WHAT SORT OF WELFARE RIGHTS PRACTICE?

Welfare rights practice can be listed under several headings:

- Casework
- Benefit take-up and publicity
- How to run a take-up campaign
- Training
- Policy advice and development
- Lobbying and campaigning.

Casework

Often the tendency is for an organisation to invest all its welfare rights resources in casework. Undoubtedly there is a huge need for casework which can pull an organisation to focus on it and casework often makes a real difference to the lives of the recipients as well as making the advice worker feel a huge sense of achievement. It is also the bedrock of welfare rights practice and any welfare rights practitioner needs to do some casework in order to maintain and develop their legal and technical skills and knowledge.

While funding is usually linked to provision of casework, it is very unlikely that there will be sufficient welfare rights resources invested to meet the full need for casework and casework alone will not adequately address problems.

For example, while casework can reveal patterns of problems – such as poor quality decision making about particular benefits, hardship caused by particular benefit rules or a local bad practice by benefit administrators, on its own, casework can seldom prevent such problems arising in the future. It is far better to tackle the underlying cause of the casework problems than simply just reacting to them.

This is why it is vital to use casework resources strategically. First, this will be to focus them on the more complex issues and on groups who may have difficulty accessing existing advice provision. It is not good use of scarce advice worker resources to have them spending time filling in benefit claim forms while people who need help with appeals are kept waiting.

Second, there should be a system for gathering examples from the problems which arise in casework. This evidence can then be used to build a body of evidence to use as a lever for change, either locally or nationally. For many welfare rights practitioners this is second sense and many agencies have mainstreamed it as part of their work (for example Citizens Advice has a long established process for this). But there are still many agencies which do not acknowledge this as a legitimate part of welfare rights practice or who do not empower and encourage their staff to operate in this way or for whom the demands of the next case feel overwhelming. As a result dreadful and preventable problems may never be brought to the attention of senior managers in benefit administering agencies.

Third, where there are specialist welfare rights staff, referral criteria must be developed in order to reduce the chances of other staff offloading all welfare rights work onto them – a recipe for overwork, demoralisation and lack of ownership by the referrers.

Fourth, identify how casework can support other organisational objectives – for example, prioritising casework services on people in rent arrears or people who receive a statutory service.

Casework also needs clear support from managers so that when the going gets tough or the other side feels hurt, the worker feels backed up and it also needs working systems.

The systems needed for casework include the following:

- Adequate reference materials and ongoing training (discussed in Chapter 3).
- Systems for recording advice given, deadlines and actions to be taken.
- Systems for following up communications with benefit providers (essential – they are too unreliable otherwise).
- One-to-one supervision arrangements. This means 'supervision' in the social care sense and when applied to advice work it 'can provide a means by which a dialogue is created, promoting self-scrutiny and challenge, enhancing professionalism development and informing the management system and, indeed the organisation's own development' (Michael Bell Associates 2000: 117). It may also be necessary to develop 'technical' supervision from outside the employing body.
- Access to more skilled and experienced advisers for help in complex cases.
- Arrangements to prevent advisers become isolated.
- Protocols for handling conflicts of interest, confidentiality and complaints.
- Quality and performance management systems (see page 107 for more on this).

Advice work has been identified as having several levels of complexity. For example:

- *Type I* – active information, signposting and explanation.
- *Type II* – casework including a diagnostic interview, making a judgement about whether or not a case can be pursued, setting out options, encouraging people to take action on their own behalf, negotiating, introducing the customer to another source of help and supporting service users to make their own case.
- *Type III* – advocacy, representation and mediation including representing at court or tribunal or complex written advocacy.

(Michael Bell Associates 2000: 7)

A welfare rights specialist would be carrying out Type II advice, a non-specialist a combination of Type I and/or II.

Benefit take-up and publicity

The scale of underclaimed benefit was highlighted in Chapter 2. There remains huge scope for improving benefit take-up and such activity is often a key part of welfare rights practice. However, the huge demand for casework can mitigate against take-up initiatives being started.

Take-up work can involve casework, telephone advice and/or written information all of which are coordinated and designed to help entitled non-claimers to make successful claims.

Experience from take-up work points towards a number of key success factors: a major key success factor is deciding whether a blanket or targeted approach will work best and being clear why a particular method is preferred. Targeted campaigns tend to have higher success rates but they reach smaller groups of people. Popular targeted methodologies include the following:

• data-matched housing benefit records to identify underclaimers
• disability and special educational needs registers
• people using particular health services, day and home care services
• residents of sheltered and supported housing schemes
• targeting by specific disability or illness where there is evidence of underclaiming among a group.

Some more imaginative examples over the years have included people formerly employed in particular occupations (e.g. former coal miners to improve take-up of benefits for work-related diseases), contacting people known to black and minority community organisations and people with sensory impairments (particularly to improve take-up of disability living allowance after positive caselaw developments).

The National Audit Office (2002) has expressed concerns that there is no standard method of measuring the impact of benefit take-up work and some benefit take-up work estimated gains rely on assumptions or do not involve actual followed up of claims in order to verify their success or failure.

There has been particularly vocal criticism by welfare rights advisers about the DWP's claimed success rates for its minimum income guarantee and pension credit take-up campaigns because there is tracking of claims made following telephone contact by the customer with the DWP and the figures for additional claims include claims generated by claimants themselves with no input by DWP as well as claims generated by the activity of other organisations.

Figures from a survey carried out by the national Partnerships Against Poverty group for England and Wales suggest that there are clearly different success rates from different take-up methodologies:

Publicity: 25% of initial contacts from publicity may go on to make successful claims. Outreach advice work: 50% of people who seek advice (bearing in mind the generally poor response rate to drop-in advice sessions which rely on people dropping in). Targeted advice work through data matching or particular customer groups . . . 80% of people targeted go on to make a successful benefit claim.

(Pension Service 2002 (Booklet 2): 6)

The authors also state:

Although a targeted approach is usually most effective, research findings highlight that entitled non-recipients are not a uniform group and that different people respond to a variety of approaches. A combined approach of publicity allied to outreach and targeted activity is therefore the most effective way to reach entitled non-recipients and to reinforce positive messages about claiming.

(Pension Service 2002 (Booklet 2): 6)

Effective publicity is also a key success factor – either as part of the campaign itself or to reinforce messages in a take-up campaign. This means that publicity must be well coordinated to fit with an overall campaign. Experience also shows that general-ised messages urging people to 'Claim it!' are of little useful effect unless they are well targeted or specify who it is that can claim it successfully or if the majority of a population qualify (which is why the approach worked well with child tax credit, with 90 per cent of families of children qualifying). This has been yet another criticism of the DWP's publicity aimed at older people which has implied that almost all pensioners qualify for pension credit. Another effect of such publicity is that high volumes of enquiries can be generated (including many claims from those who are not entitled).

Publicity which identifies who can qualify (for example, by having worked examples or case studies of known underclaimers, such as HM Revenue and Custom's working tax credit campaign aimed at single employees on modest earnings) is more likely to have an impact with groups where the numbers who are entitled is relatively small. Welfare rights advisers have also reported impressive responses to short articles about specific benefits with tear-off slips for more advice which have been placed in local authority newspapers.

Many welfare rights services also publish welfare rights leaflets which stand alone as useful, rights-based publications for the public. These include leaflets and self-help packs about issues such as how to claim disability living allowance, benefits for carers, benefits for 16 and 17 year olds, benefit rates charts, how to deal with an incapacity benefit cut-off, benefits for people in residential care, benefits and tax credits for those in low paid work (sometimes supplemented by employment rights information). Unfortunately, there is significant duplication of effort in this area with neighbouring services sometimes writing and publishing their own versions of leaflets on the same subjects.

Welfare rights practitioners have developed their own publicity materials for several reasons:

- 'Official' materials can be either too dense or simplistic to get over technical points in a succinct manner and essential rights-based messages are lacking.
- They provide an opportunity to address gaps in the publications market: can you imagine the DWP publishing a leaflet encouraging and helping people to appeal or to apply only for Social Fund grants rather than loans?
- Advice giving on social welfare law is not a value-free activity.
- They help create a climate which is more sympathetic to benefit claimants and help to counter popular myths and stereotypes about benefit entitlement. Use of local newspaper in particular – often based on human interest stories but used to branch out and 'reach' others – give claiming a positive image.

How to run a take-up campaign

Fortunately there are at least four publications which set out in some detail the features of successful take-up initiatives and all are available on their respective publishers' websites. The publications cover different methodologies and the campaign from planning through to evaluation:

- Local Government Association (1999) *It's a Right . . . Not a Lottery*. London: Local Government Association.
- Pension Service (2002) *Income Take-up: A Good Practice Guide*. London: Pension Service.
- Local Government Association (2003) *Quids for Kids: Good Practice Guide on Benefits and Tax Credits Take-up Work for Families with Children*. London: Local Government Association.
- Department for Work and Pensions (2004) *Council Tax Benefit Take-up: A Best Practice Guide*. London: Department for Work and Pensions.

Anyone thinking of running a take-up initiative would be well advised to read these publications, which draw on the experience and expertise of a large number of welfare rights professionals. *Quids for Kids* in particular addresses some of the key questions involved in running benefits take-up activity:

- What are you planning to achieve?
- Who to work with?
- Who to target? – which group(s) and which benefit/tax credits?
- How will the target group be reached?
- Is this a time-limited project?
- What follow-up work is going to be offered?
- How is the work going to be monitored and evaluated?

(Local Government Association 2003: 28)

Other issues which *Quids for Kids* highlights include how to structure any follow-up work which is to be done as part of any take-up activity and to what level the help will be provided:

- obtaining claim forms
- help with completing claim forms
- signposting enquiries to an advice service
- freepost address
- telephone helpline
- face-to-face advice – drop-in or by appointment
- home visits and
- full casework and representation service.

(Local Government Association 2003: 47)

This highlights that effective benefit take-up activity cannot occur in a vacuum and some welfare rights advice capacity may well be required to ensure it is effective.

ACTIVITY 4.2

What are the priorities for benefits take-up work?

Training

Training is not only a key element of ensuring quality and motivation among advice workers, but also an essential tool for engaging non-specialists in welfare rights work. This is why many welfare rights services have developed ongoing training programmes for people such as social workers, community nurses and housing officers. Getting others to be able to handle enquiries and make informed referrals is a good use of very scarce welfare rights resources and one which has a far bigger impact than simply passing every welfare rights problem to 'the expert'.

Good quality welfare rights training also engages people in the welfare rights philosophy and can help create a cultural change so that welfare rights activity is valued and understood. For non-experts, a welfare rights training course will typically help them to

- understand common rules of entitlement and the main exceptions to entitlement
- enable them to identify unclaimed benefits and not only to help people to claim but also to resolve problems which arise during the claims process
- empower them to resolve the more straightforward common problems – 'first aid advice and advocacy'
- make informed referrals to specialists.

Of course training alone is not sufficient – non-specialists also need access to second tier services which were considered earlier, if they are to successfully apply the training and to consolidate their learning.

Further along the spectrum, more complex welfare rights training will help people to undertake complex revisions and supersessions (particularly involving disability benefits), look at the detail of help towards housing costs, combine welfare rights training with awareness of poverty as it affects particular groups (for example, people who are sensorily impaired or who have mental health problems or people who are subject to immigration control).

Many welfare rights services within local authorities also offer training on ancillary subjects such as debt and housing rights and the rules about charges for care services.

Like advice giving, training is not a value-free activity and the interpretation of entitlement and overall approach to the work highlighted via welfare rights training is radically different from that delivered by the DWP. The latter will frequently tend to emphasise the processes involved in claiming, rely on a more restrictive view of entitlement and frequently also highlight fraud prevention.

Welfare rights training is more likely to succeed if it

- takes account of adult learning styles and involves a high level of participation and activity such as case studies
- can include some element of application after the course
- is accredited in some way and is evidenced by a certificate
- uses scenarios and explanations which are relevant to people's jobs
- avoids use of jargon and abbreviations
- is supported with good quality notes
- uses a variety of tutor styles and delivery methods
- uses case studies and other exercises to help reinforce learning
- is up-to-date and makes provision for updating
- is delivered in a lively and participative style
- is treated as a core part of the worker's job.

Frequently organisations will offer welfare rights training on a volunteer basis. While conscripts often make poor soldiers and volunteers are more likely to be engaged and interested, the lack of any sign of compulsion does mean that those who are uninterested in welfare rights practice will remain so.

Welfare rights training can act as a vehicle to changing organisational culture so that the welfare rights philosophy is accepted and staff are empowered to do welfare rights work. My enthusiasm is based on my own experiences of establishing and managing the welfare rights service in Suffolk. Each year about 1,000 person/days of welfare rights training are still delivered and a wide range of social care staff have been enabled to incorporate a realistic level of welfare rights activity in their day-to-day work. And ultimately, the service reaches far more people than if all the welfare rights work had been reserved for a small minority of experts.

Welfare rights practice also features in social work and housing professional qualifications (and the 2005 National Occupational Standards for social care workers).

But the amount of time devoted to welfare rights practice on the social work qualification varies widely because the welfare rights element does not have a sufficiently prescriptive curriculum and it is necessary to be an assessed element of the course.

Alongside training for advisers and professionals, it is also important to consider the scope for training of benefit recipients. Not only does this empower them, but also there are examples of courses being developed for long-term benefit recipients and volunteer advice workers, with the aim of enabling them to compete for jobs as paid advice workers, so helping to address the recruitment difficulties which many advice agencies face.

For paid advice workers, ongoing training is vital in an ever changing field. And it is gradually becoming a non-negotiable feature of working life. Not only are funders increasingly expecting welfare rights agencies to have training plans in place, but also it is a requirement of the two higher levels of the Community Legal Service Quality Mark and it is also an implied requirement of the emerging National Occupational Standards for legal advice in England and Wales and the Scottish Executive's competencies for debt and welfare rights advisers. Outline proposals (in the Clementi Review 2004) for formal regulation of the advice sector may well also have implications if the government takes these further.

Unfortunately, the range of qualifications in advice work is patchy – a handful of higher education institutions offer advice work qualifications and the National Vocational Qualification in Advice and Guidance is felt by many to be too generalist and does not involve technical knowledge. Inevitably paid advice workers will have to fall back on a process of continual development.

For advice workers who are also social workers by qualification, ongoing training and development is a requirement of the conditions of registration as a social worker – a process which may eventually be extended to encompass non-social worker welfare rights advisers who are employed in social care agencies.

Policy advice and development

Welfare rights advisers are well placed to comment on the impact of social security and anti-poverty policies. Indeed, they are one of the main sources of external feedback for the DWP and have a good track record in using the evidence of failure and contradictions in income maintenance policies to achieve improvements – this was discussed earlier in relation to casework. It is important that the evidence is used appropriately – for example, it is of little value lobbying the local Jobcentre Plus manager about a deficiency in the benefit rules.

However, particularly within local authorities, such activity can be viewed as low priority or as a distraction from the job. This is unfortunate because it is by changing policy and practice that major changes for the better can happen.

Welfare rights expertise can also be invaluable in ensuring that a range of services are benefit efficient. For example:

- devising strategic funding arrangements so that care home residents can access more benefits

- maximising revenue from rents in supported housing
- helping design local authority adult placement, fostering and adoption payments in a more tax credit and benefit efficient manner
- ensuring that income maximisation is built into key processes – debt collection, assessment of local authority charges, social services preventative care payments, etc.
- helping design community placement schemes which make optimum use of the benefits system as a funding stream
- advising on benefit efficient arrangements for paying service users for consultative activity
- ensuring that local authority resources are not being used to subsidise deficiencies in benefit design or delivery, for example, building in benefit checks into use of Children Act preventative payments to service users ('Section 17 money'), income maximisation for care leavers and young people in the care system.

Lobbying and campaigning

There is a certain irony that as welfare rights practice has become more mainstreamed and widespread as an activity, it has grown away from the claimant-led roots from which so much of it grew. Pressure groups and advice bodies, which involve benefit recipients as equals and in any meaningful number, are few and far between. So while welfare rights practice has become more professional, there is a danger that the very people it was designed to help, feel more excluded and disempowered by having to have an expert to act on their behalf to sort out benefit issues. While this trend is largely due to the ever growing complexity of the means-tested benefits system, it also arises because the role of claimant-based organisations has been overlooked.

There are many examples of when welfare rights advisers alongside allied professionals have linked up with benefit claimants to undertake either benefit take-up projects or to campaign about benefit issues. An example was the Towerwatch organisation in London in the 1990s which was an alliance of local authority and voluntary sector welfare rights advisers and benefit claimants who ran a successful campaign against the closure of benefit offices in London which resulted in an administrative shambles and hardship. Other examples include work done against cuts in disability benefits shortly after New Labour came to power, the activity of the National Pensioners' Convention, and work undertaken with some local centres for unemployed people.

Not only can benefit claimants be the additional people needed to make a campaign large enough to notice, but also there is a bigger public impact if a campaign involves people who are directly affected by unfair policy or legislation and who can speak directly about their experiences.

I would argue that it is a legitimate part of welfare rights practice to work alongside one's service users in efforts to change the welfare system for the better and the evidence of improvements shows that this is both achievable and desirable – the introduction of emergency payments by HM Revenue and Customs, implementation of the lower rate mobility component of disability living allowance (following lobbying by parents of children with special needs) and the special rules for disability living and attendance allowances (lobbying by hospice social workers) to name but a few.

FUNDING

Like any other service, if not adequately funded, welfare rights practice will suffer. Among non-specialist agencies, there can be a tendency to underinvest in basic necessities such as ongoing training for staff, textbooks, specialist software and access to second tier specialist advice. Textbooks in particular seem to be a common victim of false economies and the lack of sufficient up-to-date books just makes a difficult job more difficult, as well as exposing staff and their employer to the risk of complaints about misadvice. Similarly, with training there needs to be an adequate level of investment so that all non-specialists who undertake welfare rights work have access to training – five days per staff member initially with a one- or two-day refresher each year is a reasonable minimum. And despite all the knowledge and experience about welfare rights work, we still find that what passes for welfare rights training in many non-specialist agencies is to invite a local advice agency or a local DWP officer to come and give a talk at a team meeting.

For a specialist welfare rights service, funding can be a particular challenge, particularly if the organisation is small and unable to reap the same economies of scale as a larger body. External funders may have little sense of what type of service they actually want to fund and they may have only a hazy idea about the scale of need for welfare rights advice so funding often simply follows historical patterns. This syndrome is far from unknown in the public sector and achieving changes so that funding is based on a more objective footing is both organisationally and politically complex.

However, the growing expertise in commissioning of services by the public sector and the requirement to apply Best Value criteria is starting to influence funding decisions and leading funders to develop funding based on service level agreements or contracts and by increasingly specifying the outputs and outcomes which are required. The greater availability of good quality data, such as the Index of Multiple Deprivation, also enables better informed funding decisions to be made and some local authorities have commissioned external reviews of advice provision and use of software such as Michael Bell Associates' ANARAK (Advice Needs Assessment and Resource Allocation Kit) package to identify local levels of need for advice.

In recent years, many new funding opportunities have arisen for welfare rights services. This includes non-specialist agencies which employ welfare rights specialists as well as specialist welfare rights agencies within local authorities and in the voluntary sector. The list of the more common public sector funds alone is a long one:

- Direct funding by local authorities
- Legal Services Commission contracts
- Supporting People funds

- Sure Start projects
- Neighbourhood Renewal Fund
- New Deal for Communities
- Valuing People
- European Social Fund
- Primary Care Trusts
- DWP Partnership Fund
- Refugee Integration Fund
- And any number of specific grants paid to public authorities and which may be used to fund welfare rights advice for particular groups. The significant number of ring-fenced government grants that local authorities have at their disposal give them some freedom to decide how to spend, provided that they consult service users. Such consultation activity has often highlighted service users' views that welfare rights advice should be a priority area for investment.

Agencies outside the public sector will also potentially have funding from a host of charitable bodies.

The increasing reliance on such sources of funding is creating problems for the advice sector:

- Funding is usually short-term making recruitment and retention difficult and leaving gaps when funding ends. It is not unknown for advice service to have 30 per cent of their workforce funded by such schemes and the potential for poor staff morale is great.
- Each fund has different eligibility criteria and accountability arrangements, requiring a mini-bureaucracy for each one and using up manager and advice worker capacity.
- Rather than the service developing to meet a proven need, it develops in accordance with whatever external funding it can obtain – the tail wags the dog.

Part of the funding equation is of course cost. Some work has been done in individual agencies to identify the cost of advice provision – for example, the cost per enquiry or the additional benefit gain for each pound spent on a take-up campaign.

Advice agencies have particular issues, which create significant accountancy problems:

- Costs can be distorted by having unsuitable (but cheap) premises.
- Cost per enquiry can be distorted by an agency which is fortunate enough to own its own premises.
- How should one measure units of advice? In hours? Per problem asked about? Each one is deficient and, for example, the enquiry numbers which can be claimed by Citizens Advice Bureaux can mislead unless one understands their method for counting enquiries.
- When costing take-up initiatives, how far should one apportion an organisation's overheads when working out benefit return on expenditure?

- Should the costs of second tier advice agencies include an element for the work delivered by non-specialist front line staff in the same organisation?
- How should costs for resources, which are shared with non-advice agencies, be apportioned?
- How legitimate is it to count volunteer time as a hidden cost or return on an investment?
- Normal levels of staff turnover or sickness can disproportionately affect staff costs in smaller organisations.
- Is it legitimate to compare the cost of organisations which offer poorer conditions of service and which are therefore less able to attract and keep better quality staff?

While cost reduction is a legitimate part of commissioning and managing a welfare rights service, crude cost comparisons between advice agencies are unsafe and also potentially create a race to the bottom.

Some progress has been made in moving welfare rights agencies towards common methods of recording activity – though the plethora of external funding can mean that one is running more than one recording system for the same work. Performance monitoring work initiated by Leicester, Nottingham and Manchester City Councils involves requiring all funded advice agencies in these areas to adopt a common method of recording their activity and advice outcomes, differentiating the different outcomes for 'enquiries' and 'cases' as well as apportioning costs.

QUALITY AND PERFORMANCE MANAGEMENT

Closely linked to funding and cost is the whole arena of quality and performance management. And welfare rights advisers are fortunate that they are one of the few public service groups which can relatively easily measure their results – the additional amount of benefit gained from their activity is a performance measure which can also be used by non-welfare rights specialists.

Most specialist welfare rights agencies now have some form of formal quality assurance system and the most common is the Legal Services Commission's Quality Mark, which can be awarded for different levels of work. People in Scotland are spared the tedium and bureaucracy of both the Community Legal Service (CLS) and the Quality Mark.

The Quality Mark is frequently a requirement for public and voluntary funding (outside Scotland) and it is based on ensuring that an organisation has various systems in place. The systems required are generally those one would expect to find in any reputable organisation – staff and volunteer supervision arrangements, case recording systems, training plans, strategic plans, customer complaints procedures, etc. alongside some politically inspired irrelevances such as recording of referrals. However, despite the rhetoric about the Quality Mark: 'a big success story' (Lord Falconer, the Lord Chancellor, to Legal Action Group 2003 conference); 'the industry standard that assures quality advice' (David Harker, Chief Executive Citizens Advice, in Citizens Advice

2004a: 3), there remain many critics of the Quality Mark such as one delegate at the Legal Action Group's 2003 conference, who said: 'The Community Legal Service Quality Mark is a costly burden that does not measure the quality of advice given to clients' (reported in *Legal Action* January 2004).

Research among advice agencies has produced a mixed response (Braverman and Lucas 2004a: 7)

- Costs in terms of staff time for achieving a CLS Quality Mark are 'substantial' and disproportionately affect smaller organisations 'which are also more likely to be catering for socially excluded groups').
- The bureaucratic burden was less 'than had been feared' and 'once systems had been absorbed into everyday practice, they were often not perceived as a problem'.
- Most advice agencies thought the CLS Quality Mark had been useful, even though they recognised drawbacks.

The Quality Mark is linked to the Community Legal Service in England and Wales (Scotland is still spared the agonies of this New Labour initiative). There are several aims behind the CLS including improving advice standards, improving supply of publicly funded advice, moving legal aid funds into alternative advice provision and control of legal aid costs. Critics usually felt the latter is pre-eminent.

While the CLS has triggered some interesting initiatives, there is widespread concern about its effects:

- frequently moribund Community Legal Service Partnerships (with some notable exceptions)
- no long-term secure funding for core services
- a major decline in publicly funded, mainstream legal advice
- additional bureaucracy for those agencies which are funded
- exaggerated claims about the availability of effective advice provision
- awarding the Quality Mark to services, which are peripheral legal advisers, or to services which do not have the level of expertise which is claimed.

Some other quality and performance systems include the following:

- *PQASSO (Practical Quality Assurance System for Small Organisations)*: not widely used in the advice sector but some advice agencies have found that it has helped them to identify key areas for improvement. PQASSO is effectively a version of the European Foundation for Quality Management's Excellence Model which seeks to engage a range of stakeholders in helping an organisation to identify strengths and weaknesses and to improve its performance.
- *Citizens Advice accreditation*: a requirement for Citizens Advice Bureaux which involves audit of work as well as detailed procedural and other systems.
- *Chartermark*: a government award for quality public services rather than a system for performance management. Chartermarks have been awarded to welfare rights services (for example Lancashire County Council) and to services which include welfare rights advisers. Other welfare rights services have helped their local

authorities to achieve Beacon Council awards from the government (for example, Suffolk County Council for its work with young people leaving care).

- *Advice UK Achieving Excellence*: independent advice agencies can join this organisation but need to adhere to certain minimum quality standards and can work towards this quality system.
- *Quality Counts*: Age Concern's quality system.
- *DIAL UK Standards*: a system for agencies which wish to be members of DIAL.
- *Peer Review*: a process for other welfare rights practitioners to audit and comment on each other's work.

Whichever system is used, the key to success (i.e. a workable system which helps improve services) is keeping it simple and engaging staff, volunteers, managers and other stakeholders in its development and maintenance (Braverman and Lucas 2004b: 33).

The basic performance and quality system one could expect to see in a welfare rights agency (as well as non-specialist organisations) would include the following:

- A manual which contains all the procedures in one place and which is regularly updated and which users are familiar with.
- Procedures for ordering up-to-date textbooks.
- Procedures for checking, at least weekly, what developments in social security law and policy have taken place and for cascading this to others.
- A plan for ensuring that new staff are inducted and trained and that existing staff are continually developed and training needs are addressed.
- A process for checking the advice given for accuracy and completeness. Perhaps a more through audit, say annually, and possibly an accuracy score could be developed?
- Agreed time for advisers to spend discussing casework and related matters in supervision sessions and/or on a one-to-one basis with a peer.
- A workload monitoring scheme.
- A complaints procedure which includes a second stage for any complaints.
- File management and case recording processes.
- A workable system for recording the advice given (possibly copying to the customer).
- A confidentiality and data protection policy which also contains any specific exceptions (e.g. disclosure of information about risk or harm to third party).
- A strategic planning process.

Despite the criticisms of the Legal Services Commission's Quality Mark, it does at least ensure that an organisation has, at least on paper, several of the above processes.

PERFORMANCE INDICATORS

These should be useful and not an undue burden to administer (and bear in mind that they are indicators and not absolutes). But performance indicators matter because they are a way to measure success and failure and enable changes in service quality to be objectively assessed. Some indicators for welfare rights services could include the following:

- benefits gained
- debts managed
- evictions prevented
- staff and volunteer turnover and absenteeism
- days devoted to staff/volunteer training and development
- budget performance and fixed cost as a proportion of variable costs
- percentage of trustees attending at management committee meetings
- amount of computer access time
- customer satisfaction ratings
- waiting times for appointments and callers
- ethnic, gender and geographical data about customers
- percentage of maximum open time that the service is closed.

BUILDING AND SUSTAINING A WELFARE RIGHTS SERVICE

There is no getting away from the fact that welfare rights practice courts controversy. Therefore building and sustaining welfare rights practice requires clear management and political support and where welfare rights practice has become an accepted norm for an organisation, the various myths and misunderstandings about what welfare rights practice is have normally been overcome, often by regular use of performance management information and by helping any politicians see the policy linkages between welfare rights practice and their particular ideology. (For socialists and liberals, this will be that welfare rights practice encourages equality. For free marketeers, welfare rights work empowers people to be more independent and can enable the 'deserving' poor at least to be seen to be gaining. Never underestimate paternalistic Toryism!) There are also lots of practical cost-effective gains for an organisation if its staff engage in welfare rights practice which can excite even the most illiberal, financially fixated senior manager or politician. And of course it goes without saying that one can and should usually manage to actively demonstrate the ways in which welfare rights practice supports an organisation's corporate objectives.

As well as winning over converts in the easy days, it is vital to repeatedly sell the value of welfare rights work. There is much ranged against welfare rights practitioners – endless tabloid stories about welfare scroungers, nervous politicians who cannot tolerate criticism of their government's policies and ill informed decision makers who think that welfare rights advisers and benefits administrators do the same sort of work.

Writing in 1986 Fimister highlighted the necessity of getting senior managers and key local politicians on-side: 'Clear agency policy and management objectives are essential in setting the overall scene' (Fimister 1986: 39) and for welfare rights enthu-siasts to be able to influence key decision makers within an organisation:

> The political factors involved in establishing and indeed preserving a welfare rights resource are – as is the case with any policy innovation – likely to be diverse and subtle. If local welfare rights enthusiasts are to involve them-selves in creating, improving or defending such services, then these are the elements with which they must deal, learning to recognise the opportunities and pitfalls alike, to distinguish the ladders from the snakes.
>
> (Fimister 1986: 85)

Having obtained at least management support for welfare rights practice, one needs to work at ensuring that key managers' interest is maintained and they learn about some aspects of what is involved and why certain approaches are adopted. This will be particularly important when welfare rights advocacy is criticised by powerful third parties.

An engaged management style also helps ensure that welfare rights practitioners do not become isolated. Such isolation can easily occur when line managers are not particularly interested in welfare rights work and so do not understand what it involves and why. And there are too many examples of small welfare rights services being isolated, leading to introspection and often dysfunctional behaviour, the manifestations of which provide a ready excuse to shut down the service – all the more reason to constantly strive to integrate welfare rights practice into the organisation's mainstream without diluting the unique values associated with welfare rights practice.

PAY AND CONDITIONS

Pay rates for welfare rights work vary tremendously, which tends to beg questions about the so-called objectivity of the grading schemes that organisations use. Whatever the local constraints that prevail, there are some key messages about pay and conditions to bear in mind:

- An organisation developing a new welfare rights service might want to pay above the going rate in order to attract experienced advisers. An existing service may want to pay more in order to retain staff.
- The technical complexity of specialist welfare rights practice can be as challenging as any legal activity and pay rates need to recognise this.
- A salary which compares at least equally to that of other professionals in an organisation will lessen the chance of marginalisation of the welfare rights specialist and also provide opportunities for existing staff to develop by moving sideways or diagonally.
- There is a long-standing shortage of the more highly skilled welfare rights advisers and this is often the level of advice which is in short supply in an area.

- There is a case for trainee welfare rights adviser posts to ease recruitment problems and to provide opportunities for people to enter this line of work – particularly from among groups which are under represented in the workforce.

AND FINALLY . . .

Welfare rights practice is a flexible and empowering approach to helping others. It has much to offer many public and voluntary sector organisations and the people who use their services and it helps ensure better accountability of welfare bureaucracies.

While much of what I have written is drawn from personal experience over thirty odd years (some of them very odd) involvement in welfare rights practice and while some may disagree, I hope I have set out a useful framework for effective welfare rights practice by specialists and non-specialists alike.

The uniqueness and importance of welfare rights practice remain as relevant and necessary as ever. Let us wish it well.

CHAPTER 5

USEFUL RESOURCES FOR WELFARE RIGHTS PRACTICE

BOOKS AND JOURNALS

Up-to-date reference materials are the lifeblood of welfare rights practice.

TYPE I ADVICE

Not all of the following will be relevant, but 'must buys' for everyone are marked with an asterisk (*).

Disability Rights Handbook *. Disability Alliance.
Welfare Benefits and Tax Credits Handbook *. Child Poverty Action Group.
Welfare Benefits and Tax Credits CD ROM. Child Poverty Action Group.
Young Persons Handbook. Centre for Economic and Social Inclusion.
Newcomers Handbook. Centre for Economic and Social Inclusion.
Welfare to Work Handbook. Centre for Economic and Social Inclusion.
Guide to Housing and Council Tax Benefit. Shelter and Chartered Institute of Housing.
Big Book of Benefits and Mental Health. Neath Mind.
Factsheets published by Age Concern England and Age Concern Scotland.
Various guides published by Disability Alliance (e.g. *Guide to Claiming Disability Living Allowance* for children).
Student Support and Benefits Handbook: England, Wales and Northern Ireland. Child Poverty Action Group.
Benefits for Students in Scotland Handbook. Child Poverty Action Group.
Lone Parent Handbook. One Parent Families.

TYPE II ADVICE

As above, plus relevant ones from this list:

Migration and Social Security Handbook. Child Poverty Action Group.
Paying for Care Handbook. Child Poverty Action Group.
Debt Advice Handbook. Child Poverty Action Group.
Money Advice Handbook. Money Advice Scotland.
Fuel Rights Handbook. Child Poverty Action Group.
Council Tax Handbook. Child Poverty Action Group.
Child Support Handbook. Child Poverty Action Group.

TYPE III ADVICE

As above, plus the following:

Child Support Handbook. Child Poverty Action Group.
Welfare Rights Bulletin (bi-monthly). Child Poverty Action Group.
Adviser (bi-monthly). Shelter and National Association of Citizens Advice Bureaux.
Legal Action (monthly). Legal Action Group.
Disability Rights Bulletin (quarterly). Disability Alliance.
Social Security Legislation Volumes I, II, III and IV. Thomson Sweet and Maxwell.
CPAG's Housing Benefit and Council Tax Benefit Legislation. Child Poverty Action Group.

SOME USEFUL WEBSITES

The Internet is now a huge resource for welfare rights practice.

Resources for advice work

Action for Blind People: Useful resources about benefits and visual impairment: www.afbp.org
Advicenow: Accessible information about a wide range of legal rights: www. advicenow.org.uk
Age Concern England: Advice factsheets: www.ace.org.uk
Age Concern Scotland: Advice factsheets: www.ageconcernscotland.org.uk
Benefits in Mind: Neath Mind's excellent site about benefits and mental health: www.benefitsinmind.org.uk

Care and Health Law: Extremely useful site by social care and health legal framework trainer and consultant Belinda Schwehr: www.careandhealthlaw.com

Carers UK: Information about benefits and carer's rights: www.carersonline.org.uk

Centre for Economic and Social Inclusion: Useful publications and information on welfare to work issues: www.cesi.org.uk

Child Poverty Action Group: www.cpag.org.uk

Citizens Advice Adviceguide: Information about a wide range of rights (England, Scotland, Wales and Northern Ireland versions available): www.adviceguide.org.uk

Community Legal Service (England and Wales): Leaflets about a range of legal rights: www.clasdirect.org.uk

Coventry Law Centre: Rights leaflets: www.covlaw.org.uk

DFES: Education Maintenance Allowances and other iniformation: www.dfes.gov.uk

DIAL UK: Factsheets: www.dialuk.info

Disability Alliance: www.disabilityalliance.org.uk

Electronic Immigration Network: www.ein.org.uk

Ferret Information Systems: Benefits calculation and information software: www.ferret.co.uk

Greater Manchester Low Pay Unit: Factsheets about employment rights: www.gmlpu.org.uk

Immigration Advisory Service: Advice pages: www.iasuk.org

Independent Review Service: Social Fund reviews and related matters: www.irs-review.org.uk

Institute of Revenues Rating and Valuation: Housing Benefit info for advisers: www.hbinfo.org

Lisson Grove Benefits Program: Benefits calculation software: www.lissongrovebenefits.co.uk

Mencap: Factsheets: www.askmenacp.info

Money Advice Association: www.maa.i12.com

Money Advice Scotland: www.moneyadvicescotland.org.uk

National Debtline: www.nationaldebtline.co.uk

Refugee Council: Publications for advisers: www.refugeecouncil.org.uk

Rightsnet: News, discussions and resources for welfare rights work. The world's greatest welfare rights website: www.rightsnet.org.uk

Shelternet: Housing advice: www.shelternet.org.uk

Scottish Association for Mental Health: Good factsheets about benefits and mental health: www.samh.org.uk

Social Security providers

Department for Work and Pensions: On-line claim forms, legislation, guidance and other resources: www.dwp.gov.uk

HM Revenue and Customs: As above, but for tax credits: www.hmrc.gov.uk

Department for Social Development: Northern Irish equivalent of the DWP:
http://www.dsdni.gov.uk

Social Security Agency Northern Ireland: www.ssani.gov.uk

Legislation and caselaw

British and Irish Legal Information Institute: Caselaw (esp High Court and Court of Appeal) and legislation: www.bailii.org

Social Security and Child Support Commissioner's decisions: The 'official' site: www.osscsc.gov.uk

Daily Law Notes: Summaries of all cases in the higher courts: www.lawreports.co.uk

Eur-Lex: European Union legislation, caselaw and much more: europa.eu.int

Home Office: Immigration law and policy: www.ind.homeoffice.gov.uk

Her Majesty's Stationery Office: Primary and secondary legislation: www.hmso.gov.uk

Other legal resources

Infolaw Lawfinder: Searchable catalogue of UK legal materials: www.infolaw.co.uk

Law Links: On-line legal research site at the University of Kent:
http://library.kent.ac.uk/library/lawlinks/default.htm

Lexis Nexis: Some free legal resources: www.lexisnexis.co.uk

Legal resources in the UK and Ireland: Website maintained by Delia Venables: www.venables.co.uk

Other advice resources

Angus Council Welfare Rights Service: Pension Credit calculator (much better than the DWP's!): www.angus.gov.uk

Dumfries Welfare Rights: Guides and discussion board: www.welfarerights.net

EAGA: Insulation and draughtproofing grants: www.eaga.co.uk

Low Income Tax Reform Group: Advice and campaigns about tax issues affecting: people on a low income: www.litrg.org.uk

Tax Aid: Advice on tax issues for people on low incomes: www.taxaid.org.uk

Multikulti: Rights leaflets in eleven languages: www.multikulti.org.uk

Quick Calculators for pension credit, tax credits, housing benefit and income tax: www.quickcalc.net

Prescription Pricing Authority: Information and claim forms for help with health costs: www.ppa.org.uk

Some local authority welfare rights websites with useful resources

There are many, but here are a few:

Hertfordshire: www.hertsdirect.org.uk/caresupport/bnftsadvc/
Newcastle upon Tyne: www.newcastle.gov.uk/welfarerights
Glasgow: www.glasgow.gov.uk/en/Residents/GettingAdvice/WelfareRights/
Lancashire: www.lancashire.gov.uk/environment/welfarerights/index.asp
Manchester: www.manchester.gov.uk/advice/welfare/

These and many more links and resources are available at www.neilbateman.co.uk

BIBLIOGRAPHY

Abbott, S. & Hobby, L. (1999) *An Evaluation of the Health and Advice Project: Its Impact on the Health of Those Using the Service*. Liverpool: Health and Community Care Research Unit, University of Liverpool.

Abbott, S. and Hobby, L. (2000) 'Welfare benefits advice in primary care: evidence of improvements in health', *Public Health*, 114(5): 324–27.

Abbott, S. & Hobby, L. (2003) 'Who uses welfare benefits advice services in primary care?' *Health and Social Care in the Community*, 11(2): 168–74.

Acheson, D. (1998) *Independent Inquiry into Inequalities in Health*. London: The Stationery Office.

Audit Commission Housing Inspectorate (2001) *Housing Inspectorate Framework for Assessing Excellence in Housing Management*. London: Audit Commission.

Babb, P., Martin, J. & Haezewindt, P. (eds) (2004) *Focus on Social Inequalities*. London: Office for National Statistics/TSO.

Bailey, R. & Brake, M. (eds) (1975) *Radical Social Work*. London: Edward Arnold.

Baldwin, N. & Spencer, N. (1993) 'Deprivation and child abuse: implications for strategic planning in children's services', *Children and Society*, 7(4): 357–75.

Balloch, S. and Jones, B. (1990) *Poverty and Anti-poverty Strategy: The Local Government Response*. London: Association of Metropolitan Authorities.

Bateman, N. (1996) *Advocacy Skills for Human Service Professionals*. Aldershot: Arena.

Bateman, N. (2000) *Advocacy Skills for Health and Social Care Professionals*. London: Jessica Kingsley.

Bateman, N. (2004) 'Joint misadventure', *Care and Health*, 81 (14–20 September): 29.

Bateman, N. (2005) 'For whose benefit?' *Benefits*, 13(1): 45–47.

Bateman, N. and Somerville, W. (2004) *The Disability and Carers Handbook*. London: Centre for Economic and Social Inclusion.

Bebbington, A. & Miles, J. (1989) 'The background of children who enter local authority care', *British Journal of Social Work*, 19(5): 349–68.

Becker, S. (1997) *Responding to Poverty: The Politics of Cash and Care*. Harlow: Longman.

Becker, S. (2002) 'Security for those who cannot: Labour's neglected welfare principle', *Poverty*, 112 (summer): 13–17.

Becker, S. & MacPherson, S. (1986) *Public Issues, Private Pain: Poverty, Social Work and Social Policy*. London: Insight/Carematters books.

Beresford, P., Green, D., Lister, R. & Woodward, K. (1999) *Poverty First Hand! Poor People Speak for Themselves*. London: Child Poverty Action Group.

Berthoud, R., Benson, S. & Williams, S. (1986) *Standing Up for Claimants*. London: Policy Studies Institute.

Bhatia, R. & Katz, M. (2001) 'A living wage in San Francisco is associated with substantial health improvement', *American Journal of Public Health*, 91: 1396–1402.

Borland, J. (2004) *Better Advice, Better Health, Final Evaluation Report March 2004*. Aberystwyth: Citizens Advice Cymru.

Braverman, R. & Lucas, R. (2004a) *Cost of Quality Report*. London: Advice UK.

Braverman, R. & Lucas, R. (2004b) *Managing the Quality Process*. London: Advice UK.

Brewer, M. & Emmerson, C. (2003) *Two Cheers for the Pension Credit?* Institute for Fiscal Studies (IFS) Briefing Note no. 39. London: IFS.

Brewer, M. & Shephard, A. (2004) *Has Labour Made Work Pay?* York: Joseph Rowntree Foundation.

Brewer, M., Goodman, A., Myck, A., Shaw, M. & Shephard, A. (2004) *Poverty and Inequality in Britain 2004*. London: Institute for Fiscal Studies.

Brewer, M., Goodman, A., Shaw, J. and Shephard, A. (2005) *Poverty and Inequality in Britain 2005*. London. Institute for Fiscal Studies.

Brown, T. & Passmore, J. (1998) *Housing and Anti-Poverty Strategies: A Good Practice Guide*. Coventry: Chartered Institute of Housing.

Bull, D. (1982a) *Welfare Advocacy. Whose Means to What Ends?* Text of Sheila Kay Memorial Lecture. Birmingham: British Association of Social Workers.

Bull, D. (1982b) 'Social worker as advocate?' *Social Work Today*, 12(14).

Citizens Advice (2004a) *Justice Matters*. London: National Association of Citizens Advice Bureaux.

Citizens Advice (2004b) 'Health White Paper should prescribe advice', Press Release 18 November 2004. London: Citizens Advice.

Clementi, D. (2004) *Report of the Review of the Regulatory Framework for Legal Services in England and Wales* (The Clementi Review). London: Department for Constitutional Affairs.

Copisarow, R. and Barbour, A. (2004) *Self-employed People in the Informal Economy: Cheats or Contributors?* London: Community Links.

Craig, G., Dornan, P., Bradshaw, J., Garbutt, R., Mumtaz, S., Syed, A. and Ward, A. (2002) *Underwriting Citizenship for Older People: The Impact of Additional Benefit Income for Older People: A Report for the National Audit Office*. Unpublished.

Craven, T. (2000) 'Welfare rights in Liverpool City Council Housing Department', *Benefits*, 29 (September/October).

Cullen, L. (2004) 'Of little benefit', *Community Care*, 11 November.

Curtis, H. and Sanderson, M. (2004) *The Unsung Sixties*. London: Whiting and Birch.

Davies, M. (1994) *The Essential Social Worker*, 3rd edn. Aldershot: Arena.

Davies, M. (2000) *The Blackwell Encyclopaedia of Social Work*. Oxford: Blackwell.

Davies, M. (2002) *The Blackwell Companion to Social Work*. Oxford: Blackwell.

Dean, H. (2002) *Welfare Rights and Social Policy*. Harlow: Prentice Hall.

Dennis, I. and Guio, A-C. 'Poverty and social exclusion in the EU after Laeken – part 1', *Statistics in Focus*, Population and Social Conditions: Theme 3, August.

Department for Work and Pensions (DWP) (2004a) *Work and Pensions Statistics*. London: The Stationery Office.

Department for Work and Pensions (2004b) *2004 Spending Review*. London: DWP.

Department for Work and Pensions (2005) *5-year Strategy: Opportunity and Security throughout Life*. London: The Stationery Office.

Department for Work and Pensions Decision Making Standards Committee (2005) *Annual Report April 2003–March 2004*. London: DWP.

Department of Health (DoH) (1995) *Child Protection: Messages from Research*. London: HMSO.

Department of Health (2000) *The NHS Plan: A Plan for Investment, a Plan for Reform*. London: HMSO.

Department of Health (2002) *Fairer Charging Policies for Home Care and Other Non-residential Social Services – Practice Guidance*. London: DoH.

Dowling, M. (1999) *Social Work and Poverty: Attitudes and Actions*. Aldershot: Ashgate.

Edwards, S. (2003) *In Too Deep*. London: Citizens Advice.

Fimister, G. (1977) *Exceptional Needs Payment or 'Section One' Payment? The Development of One City's Policy*. Newcastle upon Tyne: City Council Welfare Rights Service.

Fimister, G. (1986) *Welfare Rights Work in Social Services*. London: Macmillan.

Fimister, G. (1995) *Social Security and Community Care in the 1990s*. Sunderland: Business Education.

Fisher, R. and Ury, W. (1981) *Getting to Yes*. London: Business Books.

Flaherty, J., Veit-Wilson, J. & Dornan, P. (2004) *Poverty: The Facts*. London: Child Poverty Action Group.

Fook, J. (1993) *Radical Casework: A Theory of Practice*. Sydney: Allen and Unwin.

Fraser of Allander Institute for Research on the Scottish Economy (2001 & 2003) *The Impact of Welfare Spending on the Glasgow Economy*. Glasgow: University of Strathclyde.

Freeman, I. and Lockhart, F. (1994) 'The reception of children into public care. What do we really know?' Paper delivered to the Association of Directors of Social Work Conference, 29 March.

General Social Care Council (GSCC) (2004) *Code of Practice for Social Care Workers*. London: GSCC.

Gilder, G. (1981) *Wealth and Poverty*. New York: Basic Books.

Goldberg, E.M. and Warburton, R.W. (1979) *Ends and Means in Social Work: The Development and Outcome of a Case Review System for Social Workers*. London: Allen & Unwin.

Gordon, D., Adelman, L., Ashworth, K., Bradshaw, R., Levitas, R., Middleton, S., Pantazis, C., Patsios, D., Payne, S., Townsend, P. & Williams, J. (2000) *Poverty and Social Exclusion in Britain*. York: Joseph Rowntree Foundation.

Greasley, P. & Small, N. (2002) *Welfare Advice in Primary Care*. Bradford: University of Bradford School of Health Studies.

Green, R. (2000) 'Applying a community needs profiling approach to tackling service user poverty', *British Journal of Social Work*, 30(3).

Griffiths, R. (1988) *Community Care: An Agenda for Action. A Report to the Secretary of State for Social Services*. London: HMSO.

Hancock, R., Pudney, S., Barker, G., Hernandez, M. and Sutherland, H. (2004) 'The take-up of multiple means-tested benefits by British pensioners: evidence from the Family Resources Survey', *Fiscal Studies*, 25(3): 279–303.

Hawker, D. (2005) 'A lot to swallow', *Community Care*, 28 April.

Higginbotham, P. (2005) *Workhouses*. www.workhouses.org.uk

Hill, P. (2004) Workshop on joint teams at National Association of Welfare Rights Advisers meeting, Blackpool, June.

Hirsch, D. & Millar, J. (2004) *Labour's Welfare Reform: Progress to Date*. York: Joseph Rowntree Foundation.

Holmes, P. (2005) 'Beyond the blame culture', *Working Brief*, February: 11–13.

Information Commissioner (2001) *The Data Protection Act 1998: Legal Guidance*. Wilmslow: Information Commissioner's Office.

Irvine, R. (1986) 'Child abuse and poverty', in S. Becker and S. MacPherson (eds) *Public Issues, Private Pain: Poverty, Social Work and Social Policy*. London: Insight/Carematters Books.

Jackson, B. & Segal, P. (2004) *Why Inequality Matters*. London: Catalyst.

Jacobs, E. (2004) 'The duties of a representative'. Paper presented to the Social Security Law Practitioners Association, May. Available on www.rightsnet.org.uk

Johnson, Alan (2004) Ministerial Statement to House of Commons, 6 December.

Kehrer, B. and Wolin, V. (1979) 'Impact of income maintenance on low birthweight, evidence from the Gary experiment', *Journal of Human Resources*, 14: 434–62.

Legal Services Commission (2004) *Causes of Action: Civil Law and Civil Justice*. London: Legal Services Commission.

Lishman-Peat, J. & Brown, G. (2002) 'Welfare rights take-up project in primary care in Wakefield', *Benefits*, 10(1): 45–48.

Lister, R. (2004) *Poverty*. Cambridge: Polity Press.

Local Government Association (1999) *It's a Right . . . Not a Lottery*. London: Local Government Association.

Local Government Association (2003) *Quids for Kids*. London: Local Government Association.

London Borough of Newham Social Regeneration Unit (2004) *Progress Report, April 2002 to March 2004*. London: London Borough of Newham.

McCarthy, M. (1986) *Campaigning for the Poor: CPAG and the Politics of Welfare*. London: Croom Helm.

McClintock, J. (1982) *The Administration of Justice for Social Security Claimants*. Sydney: Law Foundation of New South Wales (Australia).

Madge, P., Kruse, J., Twigg, P., Smith, C., Harris, F. and Wilson, J. (2004) *Debt Advice Handbook*. London: Child Poverty Action Group.

Marsh, A. & Vegeris, S. (2004) 'Employment and child poverty', in P. Dornan (ed.) *Ending Child Poverty by 2020: The First Five Years*. London: Child Poverty Group.

Mendes, P. (2004) 'Welfare lobby groups responding to globalisation', *Poverty*, 119: 11–12.

Merton Claimants Action Group (2004) www.mucw.demon.co.uk

Michael Bell Associations (2000) *Scottish National Standards and Good Practice Guidance for Housing Advice and Information Services*. Edinburgh: HomePoint.

Moss, J. (1938) *The Relieving Officer's Handbook*. London: Hadden Best.

Murray, C. (1984) *Losing Ground: American Social Policy, 1950–1980*. New York: Basic Books.

Nadasen, P. (2005) *Welfare Warriors: The Welfare Rights Movement in the United States*. New York: Routledge.

National Association of Welfare Rights Advisers (NAWRA) (2005) *Position Paper on Joint Teams*. NAWRA c/o Child Poverty Action Group, 94 White Lion Street, London, N1 9PF.

National Audit Office (2002) *Tackling Pensioner Poverty: Encouraging Take-up of Entitlements*. London: The Stationery Office.

National Children's Home (NCH) (1986) *Families Affected by Unemployment*. London: NCH.

New Policy Institute & Joseph Rowntree Foundation (2004) *Monitoring Poverty and Social Exclusion 2004*. Findings no D14. York: Joseph Rowntree Foundation.

Noble, M., Platt, L., Smith, G. & Daly, M. (1997) 'The spread of Disability Living Allowance', *Disability and Society*, 12(5): 741–51.

O'Morain, P. (2003) *Access to Justice for All*. Dublin: Free Legal Advice Centres.

Page, D. (2000) *Communities in the Balance*. York: Joseph Rowntree Foundation.

Patterson, T. (2001) 'Welfare rights advice and the new managerialism', *Benefits*, 30 (January/February).

Payne, M. (1997) *Modern Social Work Theory*. London: Macmillan.

Pension Service (2002) *Income Take-up: A good practice guide*. London: Pension Service.

Pullinger, J. and Summerfield, C. (1999) *Social Focus on the Unemployed*. London: Office for National Statistics.

Regional Centre for Neighbourhood Renewal (2004) *Local Pension Service Evaluation*. London: College of North East London.

Reith, L. (2005) 'Incapacity benefit – the end?' *Disability Rights Bulletin*, spring: 2–5.

Richmond, M. (1917) *Social Diagnosis*. New York: Russell Sage Foundation.

Ryan, M. (1996) *Social Work and Debt Problems*. Aldershot: Avebury.

Sacks, J. (2002) *The Money Trail: Measuring your Impact on the Local Economy using LM3*. London: New Economics Foundation.

Sainsbury, R. (2001) 'Getting the measure of fraud', *Poverty*, 108 (winter): 10–14.

Shaw, C. (2004) 'Interim 2003-based national population projections for the United Kingdom and constituent countries', *Population Trends*, 118. London: Office for National Statistics.

Shephard, A. (2003) *Inequality under the Labour Government*. London: Institute for Fiscal Studies.

Social Exclusion Unit (2004a) *What is Social Exclusion?* London: Office of the Deputy Prime Minister.

Social Exclusion Unit (2004b) *Mental Health and Social Exclusion.* London: Office of the Deputy Prime Minister.

Social Security Advisory Committee (2004a) *Seventeenth Report.* Leeds: Corporate Document Services.

Social Security Advisory Committee (2004b) *The Social Security (Habitual Residence) Amendment Regulations 2004*, Cm 6181. London: HMSO.

Spence, R. (2001) *Claimed It! Benefits Take-up and the Data Warehouse.* London: London Borough of Newham Social Regeneration Unit.

Sriskandarajah, D., Cooley, L. and Reed, H. (2005*) Paying their Way: The Fiscal Contribution of Immigrants in the UK.* London: Institute for Public Policy Research.

Steele, J. and Searjant, J. (1999) *Access to Legal Services: The Contribution of Alternative Approaches.* London: Policy Studies Institute.

Thomson, D. (1966) *Europe since Napoleon.* London: Penguin.

Towle, C. (1945) *Common Human Needs.* Washington, DC: National Association of Social Workers.

Townsend, P. (1979) *Poverty in the United Kingdom.* London: Penguin.

Tree, D. (1999) 'Welfare reform in the United States and the triumph of Conservatism', unpublished dissertation for Master of Arts, University of London.

Treloar, P. (2004) 'ICT and advice', *Computanews*, 134 (December).

Tunnage, B., Tudor Edwards, R. and Linck, P. (2004) *Estimation of the Extent of Unclaimed Disability Living Allowance and Attendance Allowance for People with a Terminal Diagnosis of Cancer.* Bangor: Centre for the Economics of Health, University of Wales, Bangor.

US Social Security Administration (2005) *Annual Performance Plan* www.ssa.gov/performance/2005/

Vaux, G. (2000) 'The impact of benefits advice on health', *Benefits*, 28 (April/May).

Watson, L. & Watson, N. (1986) *Planning and Managing Change.* Milton Keynes: Open University.

Wilson, R. (1993) *Unhealthy Societies.* London: Routledge.

Yeandle, S., Escott, K., Grant, L. & Batty, E. (2003) *Women and Men Talking about Poverty*, Working Paper Series No 7. London: Equal Opportunities Commission.

INDEX

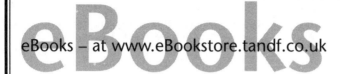